THE ANTI-AGING REVOLUTION

BREAK FREE FROM THE CHRONIC DISEASES AND
PAIN OF AGING WITH STRATEGIES THAT REVERSE
AGING, INCREASE LONGEVITY, AND ENHANCE YOUR
LIFESPAN

LISA M. WEST M.S.W. AND
JOHN J. HUMPHRIES III

CONTENTS

INTRODUCTION

NEVER TOO LATE OR TOO EARLY

It is never too late to reverse the effects of aging. All of nature and the human body can rejuvenate itself if given a fighting chance. However, to do this, you must challenge everything you ever thought you knew about aging, yourself, others, science, and the businesses and institutions that affect you daily. Since you're reading this, we are guessing you are probably a member of the Baby Boomer generation or perhaps the generation that follows, Generation X. If so, welcome—you're in the right place if you're interested in growing younger despite what "common knowledge" may be telling you. If you're not from either of the above-mentioned generations, welcome also—you are probably an enlightened Generation Z member or someone especially committed to health and wellness. It's good you're here too because aging starts sooner than you might think. Due to the lifestyles often practiced in Western cultures, doctors are now finding that our youth is suffering from diseases typically associated with aging populations, like heart disease and diabetes. The sooner you embark on an anti-aging lifestyle, the sooner you can ward off suffering from the disease of aging and the more likely you will live a long and vital life.

Chronologically speaking, we are all aging, though biologically not all at the same rate. Confronting this reality may strike fear in many of you, especially those of you who are Boomers. John and I, born at the tail end of the Boomer generation, noticed a few years ago that physically things seemed to be going downhill—fast. We were feeling less lively and more physically limited—unable to do some of the things we used to do. Our mental capabilities sometimes failed us, and often we felt we just couldn't keep up. We know that for older generations, the idea of aging can be particularly disturbing, with each generation impacted differently depending on where its individuals are in their aging journeys. We think it's fair to say that the idea of aging can be somewhat depressing for many of us.

As we age, we begin to project how life may change in the future. We may start to worry about missing the hobbies and fun things we like to do, like walking, biking, traveling, sports and games, grandkids, etc. Ultimately, we may fear isolation or the loss of independence, especially if driving a car becomes more challenging and participating in social activities gets more difficult. As we think about our own death, we may worry about leaving loved ones behind. Of course, these fears and worries only compound stress levels, which can exacerbate the process of aging and its symptoms.

Fear not! Through researching and writing this book, we gained a new perspective and personally experienced a renaissance in our own health and wellness by applying what we learned. We are especially hopeful and intrigued about how the frontiers of science are revolutionizing what we know about aging, how to combat it, and how our thinking and feeling can either promote or inhibit the aging process. In a major paradigm shift, aging is no longer seen as a collection of random diseases but as a disease itself. Consequently, some scientists believe aging can be prevented, treated, or even cured like many other diseases. Though it may be hard to believe, who knows where science may take us?

Uniquely, this book delves into evolutionary psychology about why we do the things we shouldn't and why we don't do the things we should when it comes to health and aging. Many of us live under the umbrella of not knowing what we don't know. By better understanding how we perceive the world and process information, we can recognize why we live the way we do and learn how to modify our lifestyles to improve our health and promote a vital lifespan. We can effectively achieve these goals by coupling this psychological awareness with a better understanding of the science of aging. When you get right down to it—if you want a future different from your past, you'll have to break from the past. You'll likely have to commit to making serious, personal changes in beliefs, habits, and contrary thoughts—even evaluating your support systems (family, peers, information sources, institutions, etc.).

This book takes you on a journey, not just through the psychology but also through the science of anti-aging. Though we are not anti-aging researchers, we provide you with many different lenses through which you might view the information available on the subject and a map of the territories you may choose to traverse. We will introduce you to the experts in the field so you can hear what they say about the anti-aging revolution based on the extensive research they have done. We have tried to simplify what can appear as dense scientific research and reading material into a more palatable form for our readers —in other words, there is less clinical jargon. We want you to understand how your body functions in order to appreciate the amount of stress it endures— which promotes the disease of aging and its symptoms. We hope this unique, down-to-earth presentation will encourage you to explore and gain a deeper understanding of how life impacts us at a cellular level, how our lifestyle choices impact us genetically, and how lifestyle changes and other interventions can correct and even reverse the damage done at these levels. You'll learn about remarkable studies on aging and interventions that can improve health by slowing or reversing signs of aging. Examples range from aging mice outperforming their younger counterparts to mice respectively becoming thin or obese in response to fecal matter implanted into their digestive tract from either a thin or obese human twin. We present information about octogenarians from specific cultures around the globe who demonstrate how certain perspectives and practices promote longevity and rich, fulfilling lives.

Finally, as investigators and practitioners of what we have learned, we offer a unique perspective on the positive changes we have experienced directly from the practices and interventions we have employed to improve our health and, presumably, our longevity. More details are described within, but we have seen age spots fade, hair color darken naturally, hair grow back, hip pain vanish, unwanted weight lost, improved muscle tone and dexterity, and better cardiovascular endurance. In addition to the scientific proof seen in the research studies uncovered while writing this book, the authors have lived it and experienced firsthand the benefits of a healthy lifestyle that produces anti-aging results. Approaching our 70s, we live very active and fulfilling lives. For example, we spend our time writing books, personally renovating and maintaining rental properties, regularly rehearsing and performing in a music trio, and traveling by air or with our RV camper to visit friends and family. We see only possibilities in our future and don't feel hindered by the common beliefs that you need to slow down or unduly accept the mental or physical limitations that often come with the disease of aging. To heck with that!

These personal insights and experiences are the impetus for writing this book! We hope that, like us, you are excited about gaining a new perspective that can enhance your current state of health, improve any symptoms and signs of aging, and promote a longer, more vital, and engaging lifespan. We are certain you will see and feel positive, life-affirming results if you take on the challenge because we did! Think of the rewards of a healthier and longer health span— freedom from debilitating aches and pains, mind fog, expensive medications, regular hospital visits, added stress, social isolation, etc. Not only that, wouldn't it be wonderful to experience joy and pleasure in your senior years pursuing the interests you love and

enjoying the things that bring you happiness— hobbies, social-
izing, traveling, spending time with family (especially if you
have grandkids)—without undue pain, discomfort, and worry?
Of course, it would!

Don't wait! Time is not on our side. We are losing the battle
with aging under traditional mindsets and lifestyles most of us
have practiced. The sooner we recognize the harm we are doing
to our bodies and how this promotes the disease of aging, the
sooner we will be motivated to make sweeping, healthy changes
(one step at a time) that will result in a more vital and fully
engaged lifestyle. While we recognize that everyone will have
their own anti-aging paths, it sometimes helps to know the
stories of some who have gone before...

JOHN'S STORY

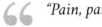 *"Pain, pain, go away... don't come back another day..."*

I was goofing around at the Jersey Shore in my early 30s when I
slipped off a skimboard and fell hard on my right hip. Even
though I knew I was injured, I had no clue what I was in for in
the long term. I was a relatively healthy young person and a
regular swimmer before my injury, so I could never have imag-
ined the painful consequences that would plague me for years.

Over time, the injury left me with chronic pain in my right hip,
which continued to worsen. It's difficult to describe to those
who have never experienced this kind of pain how it seeps into
every aspect of your life. I had to work around it constantly.

Long car rides became an ordeal. I couldn't drive a car for more than 20 to 30 minutes at a stretch, or my hip would tighten with pain. This forced me to stop periodically to stretch out my hip, a nagging reminder of my old injury. Eventually, I found that cars with cruise control provided me freedom to move my legs which offered some relief.

While walking, I realized I subconsciously changed my gait to accommodate my hip pain. Consequently, I developed a large and uncomfortable bunion on my right foot. The hip pain got so bad that I couldn't even sleep through the night. I can't remember how many nights I spent tossing and turning, trying to find a more comfortable position.

I'm sure things could have been worse, and I thank my years of regularly swimming laps for keeping my hip somewhat limber and helping with pain management. However, by my late 40s, after living with chronic pain for more than a decade, I decided something needed to change. I went to my primary doctor, who sent me to a specialist he thought could help. The specialist examined my hip and, finding no apparent cause of my suffering, sent me on my way. Before I left he offered a cortisone shot, a steroid medicine intended to reduce bodily inflammation, but it didn't reduce my pain. You could even say it made matters worse, as I now had the same hip pain as before, plus a sore injection site!

Dejected, I returned to the drawing board with few ideas for what to try next. A week passed. On the TV one afternoon, I saw a commercial featuring Regis Philbin endorsing the benefits of Osteo Bi-Flex as a dietary supplement for joint pain. The product's tagline was "Shows improved joint comfort in 7 days!"

I was intrigued, and at that point, I was willing to try anything that would help. This time, I was lucky. I still limped and had the bunion on my foot, but the supplement significantly lessened my hip pain. In addition, I didn't have to stop the car every 20 to 30 minutes when driving, and I could now sleep through the night! To this day, I still take two triple-strength Bi-Flex tablets daily (one in the AM and one in the PM), and no, this is not a paid advertisement.

In my late 50s, I noticed my hip pain started increasing again. I went back to my primary doctor and asked him to check me for signs of arthritis. My suspicions were correct. Both of my hips were affected, particularly the right. He recommended continuing with the Bi-Flex and taking ibuprofen for pain as needed. I followed his instructions, yet I continued to feel mild but nagging discomfort. Since my sleep pattern was still okay and the pain was not disabling, I resigned myself to my situation. However, I stopped taking ibuprofen because of the potential adverse side effects of NSAIDs (non-steroidal anti-inflammatory drugs).

When Lisa and I were considering writing a book about weight loss, we discovered an incredible amount of research regarding how our lifestyle choices could affect our health. In my case, I'd always had a sweet tooth and sometimes felt addicted to sugar —I often joked about being a "sugar-holic." However, I gained a little perspective after reading Ken Wilber's book, *A Theory of Everything*. I realized that sugar was indeed an addiction for me in the classic sense: I was eating it as comfort food to soothe myself when I felt lonely or sad. Essentially, I ate sugar to satisfy emotional and physiological cravings and not simply for an enjoyable experience. Our society's aggressive marketing of products containing sugar and simple carbs only encouraged my habit.

Family and holiday get-togethers always involved an array of sweets, which added to the temptation. On the flip side, my scientific background made it hard to ignore the health consequences of eating sugar, from promoting inflammation to increasing cancer risk. Based on a greater understanding of how my perspective influences my health choices and from our study of the scientific research, I decided to quit eating sugar cold turkey. What this personal experience suggests to me is that with a fresh outlook on health and aging it might be easier to fully embrace the numerous opportunities science and technology have to offer.

LISA'S STORY

 "Your body has an amazing ability to heal when given a chance."

Like John, I underwent a long journey that ultimately changed how I viewed aging and its associated health problems. As a child, I had no doubt I would live a long and healthy life since most of the older relatives I knew growing up lived into their nineties, some without any real health problems.

I considered myself an athletic child and young adult. I rode horses and took ballet classes when I was very young, and later in college I was a part of a modern dance group. When I got married, my husband at the time supported me in opening a health club. Like any business, serving my clientele was always on my mind, and my members were always asking about losing weight. So, I added a weight loss program to the club's offerings. I picked Biometrics, a 6-week heavy weightlifting program coupled with a lower-calorie meal plan.

My parents, who were in their 70s and lived nearby, decided they wanted to lose weight and get fit. Despite being relatively healthy, they were both starting to feel the effects of their age. My mother had begun to stoop and had a limp when she walked from what I believe was plantar fasciitis. Her doctor wanted her to have foot surgery, which she kept putting off (thank God, as you will see). I was thrilled they wanted to get healthier but concerned about the rigorous weight training part of the program.

About 4 weeks into the Biometrics program, I remember looking up from where I stood at the front desk at the gym and seeing my mother. She had come in early to walk on the treadmill as a warm-up for the Biometrics weight training session. All at once, I realized something incredible; she was no longer stooping or limping! It seemed the pain from her plantar fasciitis was gone. It was amazing—she looked tall and strong as she walked briskly on the treadmill. I thought she looked statuesque. This transformation only took four weeks. Even though I was familiar with the program, I was pleasantly surprised at the results she had seen in such a short time, mainly because she was in her seventies. I had thought it would take much longer to see improvements at that age. At that point, I became convinced that the human body can rejuvenate quickly under the right circumstances, even at an older age.

Years later, I retired from the fitness business, and since being healthy was no longer a job requirement, I began to slip in my diet and exercise routines. I was not taking care of my health the way I used to, and when I reached my 60s, it really began to show. I couldn't keep my weight at a healthy level, and my cholesterol was rising, too. I knew the dangers of these health issues, but my attempts to lose weight ended in disappointment. At last, I took up a medically supervised weight loss program, one I had previously been certified to teach as a health educator while working for an endocrinologist. The program used pre-packaged food and prescribed burning at least 300 calories daily from added exercise. That's a lot.

The pre-packaged meals suited me as I'm not especially fond of cooking and kept me within my 1200-calorie-a-day allotment while also preventing hunger. I had confidence in the program; after all, I had helped many obese patients lose weight on it. As expected, after 4 ½ months, I had lost 25 pounds and started to feel great about my health again. I realized firsthand the tremendous difference losing weight can have on your health. And, as you'll soon discover, it will also make you younger!

Still, something was amiss. I couldn't live on vacuum-packed meals with a year-long shelf life. I was sick of them. And the protein shakes that were part of the program were packed with saccharin, which I later found out can adversely affect the gut microbiome, causing inflammation. So, I started researching alternatives, thinking about designing a program of my own and maybe even writing a book. As health and fitness are priorities in John's life, he joined me in my research. It wasn't long, however, before what we initially intended as a weight loss guide became much more expansive.

THE TURNING POINT

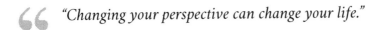 *"Changing your perspective can change your life."*

The turning point came with the discovery that maybe our focus was too narrow. We had been keeping up with the latest research on health and wellness, and, as mentioned earlier, we were thinking of compiling a book on new and effective ways that people could lose weight. However, it wasn't until we began to understand the biological and genetic benefits of weight loss that we discovered that these biological and genomic processes were the key to fighting aging itself.

This gave us the inclination to delve into research on aging and anti-aging. What we found seemed unbelievable: the possibility that aging could be slowed or even reversed. Dr. David Sinclair put out cutting-edge scientific research to this effect, while Drs. Robert Wallace and Steven Gundry report fascinating discoveries on how the gut microbiome affects one's health and ultimately how one ages. Finally, we discovered the book *The Blue Zones* by Dan Buettner, which investigates the cultures of the longest-lived people in the world, revealing that they all had several lifestyle practices in common.

Speaking of lifestyles, here in the U.S., obesity has become an epidemic. In fact, in 2021, the Centers for Disease Control (CDC) reported that 42.4% of Americans were dealing with obesity between 2017 and 2018. That percentage rises sharply to 73.6% when you factor in overweight Americans who don't qualify as obese. Further, obesity can increase the risk of, or worsen, many diseases linked to aging, from heart attacks to stroke, high blood pressure, type II diabetes, reduced pulmonary function, and more. *You could even say that the obesity epidemic is causing our population to age prematurely.* According to 2019 data from the CDC, "Life expectancy for the U.S. population in 2019 was 78.8 years." It only increased one-tenth of a year (just a little over a month) from 2018, a sad statistic considering the rapid advances we have seen in science, medicine, and general knowledge about health and wellness. As it turns out, perspective matters when practicing health and wellness.

During our research, we (John and I) were both undergoing our health journeys and were realizing how our perspectives on aging influenced our lifestyle choices in ways we may not have recognized before. Armed with our new knowledge and understanding, we set out to make more fundamental changes to our lifestyle. Nothing was safe from the microscope. We changed how we thought about aging, affecting what and how often we ate, what supplements we took, and our exercise routines. Thanks to our new mindset, diet, and intermittent fasting regimen, we both dropped 25 pounds within five months, with John reaching his lowest weight in decades. Not only that, John's inflammatory pain in his hip began to decrease as soon as he cut sugar from his diet! He noticed a change within a matter of days, and after two months, he had barely any pain at all. As of this writing, he is pain-free.

The improvement in our health has been astounding. Not only are we in better health now, but we also believe we've increased our "health spans" and longevity. *Health span*, a term that will become very important in this book, is the length of time in a person's life when they are not just alive (which is referred to as lifespan) but living a healthy and active life. Increasing our expected health spans has been a gift of immeasurable value, inspiring us with the prospect of more quality time to spend with each other, family, and friends, and contributing our time, talents, and experience to the endeavors about which we care. The research we've discovered and the efficacy of the habits we've adopted have blown us away. We wrote this book to share the benefits of what we've learned so others can take heart, learn, and benefit from a long, healthy, and satisfying lifespan.

Through writing this book and seeing improvements in the quality of our health, I (John) couldn't help but notice a correlation with the progress made in environmental health in the United States. During my 27-year career at the U.S. Environmental Protection Agency, I saw firsthand how regulatory influences brought about positive changes in air and water quality in the United States. It took a couple of decades, but environmentally conscious corporate behavior improved air quality. In addition, restored water bodies once dead from extensive chemical pollution became viable habitats for a diverse community of living creatures and plant life. Have you recently seen big headlines about smog in Los Angeles, CA, or the negative impacts of acid rain on the surfaces of buildings, crops, and plant life? It's unlikely that you have recently, although those used to be pressing issues. Also, remember how the human reduction of chlorofluorocarbons (CFCs) helped reduce the size of the hole in the protective ozone layer of the Earth's atmosphere. Even though these specific environmental issues are largely mitigated, they continue to be issues that need attention, just like other environmental threats, like global warming, fracking, and indoor air pollution.

My observations suggest that with a bit of help and assistance, the environment can recover from adverse circumstances resulting from abuse and neglect. Like the environmental restoration I observed, similarities exist in the restorative powers of the human body. This is not really a big leap since we are, in essence, an integral part of the natural ecosystem. The ills and chronic disease symptoms from years of neglect and abuse can often be reversed or mediated if more healthy choices and behaviors are selected and practiced daily. One typical example is how lung health can improve when long-time smokers quit smoking and give their bodies a fighting chance to recover and improve. All kinds of health conditions can improve with a healthy lifestyle, like heart and cardiovascular health, pain, inflammation, cancer risks, skin quality, physical strength, stamina, etc. Like the old computer analogy "garbage in, garbage out," what we feed our bodies can influence their performance. Will we choose to nurture a healthy body or allow ourselves to become an ill-fated organism destined to decline quickly over time? If we give our bodies a chance with our daily health choices, the troublesome symptoms of age-related diseases could be avoided or even reversed given time.

So, what was once supposed to be a book about weight loss is now about fighting the disease of aging and the new tools that are rapidly becoming available. This book crosses over into a new paradigm where dying may no longer be an absolute but just an untreated consequence of the disease of aging.

If it sounds like the stuff of science fiction, read on. Many leading research scientists are drawing these same conclusions. It's all a matter of perspective, as you will see.

PART I: PERSPECTIVE MATTERS

 "The body achieves what the mind believes..."

— ANONYMOUS

PERSPECTIVE AND OUR AGING DESTINY

In order to explain how we all come to frame our own unique perspectives on life, we decided to draw concepts and ideas from Ken Wilber's book *The Theory of Everything*. Wilber's concepts allow us to examine our mindsets about aging and consider the pros and cons of how we think regarding our own health and well-being. A range of cultural and social factors play into a person's opinions in every aspect of life. Using Wilber's concepts, you can help yourself become aware of these influences and objectively analyze your thoughts. This objective analysis can help you decide whether your attitudes on aging are conducive to a healthy anti-aging lifestyle or whether you need to look beyond your current horizon.

Wilber's book plays on the concept of the "theory of everything" in physics: A theory that would unite all the bits and pieces of scientific knowledge humanity has accrued, supposedly explaining everything there was to explain about the universe. In his introduction, Wilber remembers with a wry fondness the burgeoning rumors of the theory of everything as they emerged in the 80s and 90s, recalling how people would whisper that the theory of everything would show "the very hand of God in its formulas" or that the "veil had been lifted from the face of the ultimate Mystery" (Wilber, 2001).

The whisperers Wilber references talked about string theory, also known as M-theory, which attempts to unite all models of physics into an "all-encompassing supermodel." The model presumes that tiny vibrating strings make up the universe, the frequencies of which determine the nature of each and every aspect of the universe and the way everything interrelates. While M-theory shows great promise, it has yet to be proven and may not be for a very long time, if at all.

Wilber points out a couple of issues with the idea that M-theory would explain everything, expressing doubt that the vibrations of these strings could explain the subjective parts of the human experience, such as music, art, wonder, and love. He suggests that a more expansive theory is necessary, one that takes "matter, body, mind, soul, and spirit" into account. He attempts to present an "integral" approach to understanding our existence in his book (while acknowledging that the result will necessarily be imperfect!). Utilizing Wilber's concepts gives us a more holistic perspective on our lives and choices, opening up a world of new possibilities, including a longer, healthier, and more satisfying lifespan.

We will look at two parts of his theory—levels of development and quadrants. Levels of development are both personal and cultural lenses through which we perceive, while quadrants outline who or what may influence our perspective from the information they provide.

This dynamic interplay between levels of development and quadrants creates a framework for how we see life and what is possible. We hope the following discussion will give you a more expansive look at influences in your life and thus broaden your perspective, especially regarding aging and longevity.

THE LEVELS OF DEVELOPMENT

One of the earliest concepts Wilber introduces in his book *A Theory of Everything* is the eight "Levels of Development." These Levels of Development were inspired, in part, by Don Beck's and Chris Cowan's book, *Spiral Dynamics: Mastering Values, Leadership, and Change*. One of Wilber's basic concepts is this: Different people operate on different levels of awareness, and those on different levels experience reality differently. While this idea might sound a little "out there," it is drawn from the field of developmental psychology and the conclusions of hundreds of researchers therein. Developmental psychology examines the development and evolution of consciousness over time. While there are many disagreements regarding the details, the field seems to agree on one major thing—that the development of human consciousness can be modeled as a series of stages, waves, or steps. Wilber cautions the reader to remember that development is not a rigid march from one stage to the next and that people may fluidly move between levels. For this reason, he does not characterize the movement between stages as rungs up a ladder but as a spiral.

The book proposes that each individual can access any of these memes or levels. We can deepen our awareness of how humans interact with each other and the world by understanding from which levels people are operating. The first six levels are referred to as "subsistence levels." The final two are called "being levels" and represent a second tier of thinking.

Before delving into the Levels of Development Wilber describes, we'd like to reiterate that it's entirely possible to incorporate beliefs from more than one level; in fact, doing this is characteristic of the more evolved *being* levels. For instance, a person who operates in one of the *subsistence* levels believes they have the "correct" viewpoint. In contrast, a person operating from one of the *being* levels understands the need for a more inclusive perspective, one that allows us to step back, understand, and incorporate aspects from other levels as needed. With this in mind, let's look at the different levels.

Beige (Archaic-Instinctual)

At this level, the individual's only major priority is day-to-day survival. They operate on a level primarily dictated by instinct and habit, and their main concerns are the basics necessary for life. Social groups form around working with others to fulfill these needs. Wilber calls these "survival bands."

Purple (Magical-Animistic)

At this level, the individual has concerns beyond their basic needs and has the time and ability to contemplate themselves and the world around them. The idea of spirituality emerges, involving spirits who not only affect the world and its events but also govern bonds between individuals. Social groups and political connections form around concepts like ethnicity, kinship, and lineage, as does the individual's sense of identity.

Red (Power Gods)

Here, we see the development of an awareness of self that is not entirely linked to an individual's connection to their social group, family, or tribe. Instead, a sense of individuality and a distinct "self" appears. The self may be impulsive and egotistical, desiring power or glory. The concept of deity emerges, and the world is thought to operate under the influence of powerful forces, which can be either helpful or dangerous. This paradigm comes through very strongly in tales of mythological heroes, where a glory-seeking protagonist traverses an unpredictable world ruled by fickle gods.

Social groups form around the need for protection and leadership in such a world. Here we see the emergence of kings and queens, feudal lords, dictators, gang bosses, and other absolute rulers that protect their followers in exchange for obedience. Labor is performed in service to the leader.

Blue (Mythic Order)

At the fourth level, a direction or purpose to life emerges based on an all-powerful "Order" or "Being." This omnipotent entity is the source for establishing rules, hierarchy, and definitions of right and wrong. This same force defines the consequences of people's actions, good or evil, and enforces them. The establishment of rules may be attributed to a religious figure, such as a creator god, or a secular "mission" or way of thinking. In other words, the rules are no longer based solely on the whims of a living human leader but on some greater authority. People's roles in life and what's expected of them are derived from their place in the predetermined social hierarchy. The hierarchy dictates that certain people be given power over others due to the established code or rules rather than by consensus or merit. Those in positions of authority may have a paternalistic attitude toward those on lower levels. Conformity is rewarded, while deviance is punished.

Orange (Scientific Achievement)

The fifth level is significant because the individual's ability to seek an objective truth for themselves is acknowledged for the first time. Shifting from the "top-down code of conduct" of Blue and the "submission to a leader for protection" of Red, the person at the Orange level examines the world experimentally and seeks an objective understanding of how it works based on rational, mechanistic natural laws. Objective understanding explains how people and political and social groups interact. People at the Orange level view people's roles and relationships in terms of objective achievement or merit. Consequently, by virtue of varying levels of education, abilities to strategize, or expertise, some people at this level will rise above others, creating a natural hierarchy based on achievement.

Green (Sensitive Self)

In this last subsistence level, the individual expands their point of view beyond the cold rationality of Orange or the mandatory obedience of Blue and Red and begins to incorporate concepts such as empathy, sensitivity, and kindness to all into their code of conduct. Value is ascribed to individuals simply because they are alive, not because of their achievements or adherence to a set of rules. Personal bonds such as family, friendship, and love are valued over social hierarchies. Association with communities is based on shared ideas and values. Spirituality may once again become valued in contrast to the Orange stage, and the individual begins to appreciate dialogue, understanding, consensus, and harmony between groups. Social awareness, sensitivity, and multiculturalism appear for the first time.

Yellow (Integrative)

In the first of the two "being" levels, the individual incorporates hierarchical and egalitarian attitudes from all previous levels to form a more integrated viewpoint. While they value egalitarianism and fair treatment, they also acknowledge personal achievement and how, in some situations, ranks will naturally develop. When it comes to leadership from this viewpoint, a person's ability, competence, and knowledge about the issue at hand are valued over assigned hierarchies. This individual is aware of the fluid mix or spiral of levels/memes/perceptions of varied and dynamic realities, and the individual acknowledges that people can and will move between them. Nested hierarchies based on functionality, flexibility, and spontaneity emerge in institutions.

Turquoise (Holistic)

This is, perhaps, the ultimate level to strive for, or the rumored "theory of everything": A unification of all previous levels that results in a complete understanding of the universe and the nature of existence, including feeling and intuition. This results in a fluid and dynamic universal order rather than one based on rules, group bonds, or social hierarchies.

In conclusion: Each of these various levels of development are lenses through which we view the four areas of human existence, which Wilbur calls "quadrants." It's helpful to understand the nature of each of the four quadrants and the type of information they provide, but remember, the levels of development determine how we process that information. For example, the information we might receive from our family may differ from what the latest science tells us about healthy eating. Your lifestyle choices and how well you age will be based on your level of development and the sources of information you feel you can trust. Now, let's look at these four quadrants of human existence for a broader view of the information sources that can influence you and, ultimately, your health choices.

THE FOUR QUADRANTS OF HUMAN EXISTENCE

As just discussed, each quadrant can influence our thoughts, beliefs, opinions, and actions for better or worse. So, as you move through the list, think about the influence of each quadrant in your own life!

Quadrant 1 ("I" Space–Intentional)

Who are you, in your own eyes? What do you value? What do you think of the world around you? What experiences do you have that inform your inner understanding of yourself? Every person has a self-image that affects their relationship with others and the world. The first quadrant of human existence concerns a person's awareness and understanding of their beliefs, values, and experiences. For example, a person might feel afraid of aging and struggle to process their mortality, no longer having the ability to do the things they enjoy, and losing their independence. On the other hand, a person might feel more positively about aging, seeing it as another life stage they look forward to experiencing in a long and healthy old age. "Knowledge" in the first quadrant encompasses knowing what you think and feel, thus influencing your choices and actions.

There are numerous ways you can refine your awareness in the first quadrant. People work on their inner awareness by engaging in introspection, contemplation, and reflection, as well as through more spiritual means such as prayer. In addition, meditation, yoga, and breathwork can be used as tools to advance one's self-awareness. In some cultures, people have found psychedelic drugs and "plant medicines" helpful in experiencing a more profound understanding or realization of themselves.

How might you expand your understanding of aging in this first quadrant? Many people have preset beliefs about aging that they have never fully examined. Examples of limiting thoughts that might arise are, "It's too late for me to combat aging," or "Nothing can be done anyways." Engaging in contemplation can help you explore your beliefs about aging, allowing you to discard unhelpful or limiting ideas. This leaves room for more life-supporting perspectives that can open up new opportunities for you to accept where you are but also recognize how you may be able to stop or reverse aging and enjoy more of life. More specifically, ask yourself, "How would my outlook on life change if I knew I would live to 103?" Asking this question may illicit thoughts or reflections on aging and your life that may not have been otherwise available or considered. How would your view of your career, family, finances, health, and retirement change?

Throughout the book, we will refer to Quadrant 1 as the collection of the individual's personal beliefs, understandings, and experiences.

Quadrant 2 ("We" Space–Cultural)

Have you ever heard someone express a social or political opinion that most consider hateful or offensive, only for someone else to excuse their comment by saying, "They're from a different time," or, "That's just the way they were raised"? When someone points out an individual's background as a reason they hold certain beliefs, they're referencing the second quadrant of human existence. The second quadrant concerns how our families, cultural backgrounds, peer groups, and other social environments influence our thoughts, beliefs, and behaviors. It also includes messaging from the media a person consumes, be it entertainment, advertising, propaganda, or the news. Often, we're unaware of how these social forces influence and have a lasting effect on how we see things. Like other areas of life, social or cultural norms influence a person's beliefs about aging.

These beliefs can be positive or negative. Some belief systems encourage their adherents to remain healthy and treat disease and infirmity whenever possible. Others encourage their followers to accept aging as an unavoidable part of life. Certain religions include a belief in an afterlife where people's youth and health are restored. These sentiments can seem like a given to people steeped in a particular religious or cultural context, making it harder to examine these beliefs objectively.

There's nothing inherently wrong with holding beliefs from your social, religious, or cultural experiences. However, examining the pros and cons of these beliefs may be valuable. Regarding aging, unearthing a more complete understanding of your beliefs may encourage adopting new ideas and anti-aging behaviors.

Throughout the book, we will refer to Quadrant 2 as the collection of family, community, and cultural influences.

Quadrant 3 ("It" Space–Behavioral)

Imagine two people who scroll through social media while drinking their morning coffee. Both people spot the same article praising a brand-new lifestyle change that is said to restore strength to aging muscles. Perhaps the article suggests incorporating a particular ingredient into your diet. The first person is very skeptical of this claim but spots that there is a scientific paper referenced in the article. They find the paper and give it a read-through, discovering that the sample size was very small and that the results were not as conclusive as the article led them to believe. Therefore, they decide not to make this lifestyle change. The second person in this scenario is less familiar with how science is conducted. However, seeing that the article says a scientific paper supports its claim, they pick up the ingredient on their next shopping trip.

While the scenario above is fictional, it demonstrates the impact of the third quadrant, which is how scientific research and other substantiated information influence the individual. People have different levels of *scientific literacy*, which is the individual's knowledge of science and their ability to discern evidence, interpret data, and explain conclusions in a scientifically sound way. Understanding the scientific process is just as important to scientific literacy as knowing scientific facts, as it allows individuals to evaluate the veracity of claims they encounter in their daily lives.

Knowledge is power; therefore, to expand your awareness in the third quadrant, it's essential to educate yourself about how science works and what the current research on aging suggests. If you need help getting started, there are numerous guides online about how to read and interpret scientific articles and spot trustworthy and untrustworthy sources.

Throughout the book, we will refer to Quadrant 3 as the collection of scientific and technological influences on our lives.

Quadrant 4 ("Its" Space–Social)

Imagine this scenario: An individual in their 60s goes to their regular doctor for a checkup. They tell their doctor they've been dealing with persistent hunger and thirst, tingling in their hands and feet, and feeling sluggish. After undergoing tests and waiting for results, this person finally gets an answer. They're experiencing insulin resistance, one of the warning signs of prediabetes and type 2 diabetes. So, the doctor suggests this person make some lifestyle changes, such as cutting sugar out of their diet as much as possible and getting regular exercise. The doctor offers additional educational resources and also gives the patient a booklet of information on insulin resistance and how best to manage it.

In the following weeks, this person is, fortunately, able to get support from the institutions around them. For example, they have access to a nearby grocery store and can stock up on vegetables and healthy fats to build meals around. In addition, their city's infrastructure and layout make it easy to walk to work, and they can exercise at available parks and other public spaces.

Modern society is made up of an incredible number of institutional systems, more than ever before. These systems are so numerous, interconnected, and normalized that the average person is only vaguely aware of how many they interact with each day. A few examples include federal, state, and local governments, utility companies, the justice system, infrastructure and city planning, religious institutions, the healthcare system, education, and local businesses. The fourth quadrant focuses on systems and institutions that affect the quality of what's available to us daily. By supporting or rejecting certain policies, funding or cutting funding to specific projects, or adopting or rejecting new technologies, institutions can have a massive effect on whether the people who live within them can make healthy lifestyle and medical choices.

Consider the example above. This person was somewhat fortunate. The institutions around them made it relatively easy to make healthy lifestyle changes to combat their insulin resistance. But if this person did not have access to support from the institutions and systems around them, it would have been more challenging for them to make the lifestyle changes recommended by their doctor. We can better assess how much support is available by looking into various institutions and systems in our lives. To increase your awareness of the institutions and systems at your disposal, you can read about your local government, healthcare system, and other institutions. As you assess them, you could ask yourself, "Are they supporting healthy lifestyle choices, do budget cuts limit them, or are they cost-prohibitive? What efforts are being made to educate the population?" Finding answers to these questions can tell you whether the systems you live within positively or negatively affect your ability to make informed, healthy choices.

Throughout the book, we will refer to Quadrant 4 as the collection of corporate, governmental, and institutional influences.

WHY DOES IT MATTER?

How does a discussion about human levels of development and quadrants of information apply to how we deal with aging? Overall, every Level of Development involves tendencies that could be beneficial or detrimental when it comes to health and embracing anti-aging interventions. For example, those within the Purple (Animistic-Magical) level are likely to value the wisdom that comes from age and, as a result, may want to live longer. However, a strong belief that spiritual forces determine life outcomes can reduce a person's likelihood of embracing scientific advancements (Quadrant 3). On the other hand, people operating under the Green (Sensitive Self) paradigm, where empathy and understanding are the goals, are likely to stand behind progressive social programs (Quadrant 4) that aim to educate the public on healthy lifestyles or provide access to medical treatments. However, the value they place on dialogue and consensus can be crippling to advancement if everyone can't agree on the right way forward.

From this discussion, we can see that a person's Level of Development plays a significant role in how they process and act on the information they receive from the four quadrants, especially regarding how they think about aging and anti-aging interventions.

Given that most people desire to live as long and as well as possible, it makes sense to utilize a framework that explains why we often act in ways that are not always in our self-interest, especially regarding health and wellness, and why we sometimes avoid things that could be beneficial. For example, why are over three-quarters of the U.S. population overweight or clinically obese? What is influencing us, and from where does it come? To illustrate and clarify this point, let's look through the lenses of two of the most prominent (populated) levels of development and see how each of these perspectives could influence what information is sought, considered, and ultimately used. We do this with the understanding that people who occupy each of these paradigms are also three-dimensional individuals who draw from various opinions within their worldviews.

PART II: TWO PROMINENT
PERSPECTIVES

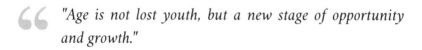 *"Age is not lost youth, but a new stage of opportunity and growth."*

— BETTY FRIEDAN

In his discussion about the Levels of Development in *A Theory of Everything*, Ken Wilber notes approximately how many people he estimates operate within each level. He suggests that about 40% of the Earth's population views the world through the Blue paradigm, while another 30% views the world from the Orange paradigm. Given that there are at least eight defined Levels of Development, that's a lot of people operating just within these two! However, these two paradigms are incredibly different, and, as a result, they see the issue of aging and anti-aging very differently. Since the life perspectives of these two ways of thinking are so common yet so different, we've chosen to take a more detailed look into their views on aging. We aim to illustrate how deeply one's Level of Development can affect their thought process and decision-making.

Though people with Blue and Orange perspectives often hold vastly different opinions on aging, they also may agree in some unexpected ways, though for different reasons. First, we'll look at how people with the Blue perspective might see the different quadrants, and then we'll see how people with the Orange perspective may see the same quadrants.

THE BLUE PERSPECTIVE OF THE FOUR QUADRANTS

Quadrant 1 – *Personal Beliefs/Understandings/Experiences*

In the Blue perspective, there is an outside Order that predetermines outcomes and ordains the rules of existence. Because of this, people who think in the Blue way tend to believe aging is inevitable and natural. Because they believe that the Order enforces consequences and rewards for people's behavior, they may also believe that this Order may bless them with a longer and healthier life if they are faithful to the prescribed code of conduct. They may also believe eternal life awaits them after death, where the Order will restore their youth and strength. This belief can bring people who subscribe to it a lot of comfort regarding aging and mortality. This peace of mind can help them manage stress as they age and thus have a positive effect on their health and well-being.

Quadrant 2 – Family/Community/Cultural Influences

Social expectations to live in the way laid out by the Order is a significant part of the Blue perspective. People at this level of development tend to follow the norms of their social group when it comes to aging and other topics, as they believe this is the key to success and happiness. Nonconformity can be met with consequences such as being socially ostracized. People within the Blue level may also be open to faith healing or other "miracle cures" if the Order they believe in endorses these measures. On the flip side, they may be suspicious of scientific advancements, new medical interventions, and anti-aging innovations if their group does not endorse them. Alternatively, the code of conduct they subscribe to can have a positive, helpful influence on their health choices. For example, there is a comfort in knowing the rules and expectations of behavior that the Order prescribes. Adherence and, thus, acceptance could foster high self-esteem and security. This may lead to lower stress levels, which is psychologically and physiologically beneficial. Whether their social group supports medical interventions or not, people at the Blue level of development are more likely to look to their code of conduct for guidance when making health decisions rather than individually evaluating available scientific data.

Quadrant 3 – Scientific/Technological Influences

People with the Blue perspective believe that the Order ordains life outcomes, so they may be reluctant to try new medical interventions that alter their bodies or extend their lifespans.

Likewise, scientists and researchers at this level of development may be unwilling to delve into areas of research they believe will interfere with the Order's plan or intention for humans, for example, DNA reprogramming or stem cell research. This attitude can be limiting when it comes to advancing scientific understanding of aging and how to combat it.

Quadrant 4 – Corporate/Governmental/Institutional Influences

Many institutions worldwide operate from the Blue perspective while applying current science to health and aging. Two examples of these institutions may be religious organizations or governments (especially state or local) with conservative leanings. Religious organizations and the clergy representing them may guide their adherents on acceptable medical interventions. Government institutions that have a Blue perspective may take steps to enforce the code of conduct they believe the Order has set out. They may do this by choosing not to fund research in certain areas or limiting access to interventions, for example, legislating against comprehensive women's healthcare or expanding Medicare coverage.

THE ORANGE PERSPECTIVE OF THE FOUR QUADRANTS

Quadrant 1 – Personal Beliefs/Understandings/Experiences

People at the Orange level of development agree that aging is natural and that everyone dies eventually, not because of a preordained Order but because of the biological processes that drive aging and death throughout the natural world. They would go on to say that since we can learn about the laws of nature and how to manipulate them to our benefit, we can and should use science to extend and improve our lives. They will likely read up on what lifestyle changes promote good health and longevity and whether they are scientifically supported.

Quadrant 2 – Family/Community/Cultural Influences

People who operate within the Orange perspective see following the current scientific and medical recommendations as the best way to care for themselves. They tend to get care for themselves when they're sick, get regular checkups, seek medical advice when they're unsure about something, and so on. As they see nature as a "well-oiled machine," they tend to view taking care of their bodies like regular maintenance of their car—the responsible thing to do to stay in top shape. Just as they would want a qualified mechanic to fix their car, they prefer the most skilled doctors, nurses, dietitians, and other medical professionals when getting advice or treatment. They respect the recommendations of physicians and researchers who are successful in their fields and are suspicious of those making unscientific claims or promoting non-scientific interventions, such as faith healing or homeopathy. Since fitness, competitiveness, youth, and attractiveness are all very important to people at the Orange level of development, they are more likely to choose any intervention that science suggests will help them stay young and healthy.

Quadrant 3 – *Scientific/Technological Influences*

Many scientists are at the Orange level of development, and these researchers tend to view age-related diseases as a collection of individual disorders they can tackle by applying scientific knowledge to develop interventions. From this perspective, the scientific method is the best way to determine what works and doesn't to combat age-related diseases. However, since the Orange perspective struggles to integrate viewpoints outside the current scientific paradigm, Orange scientists can get stuck in a rut investigating these disorders separately instead of looking for ways to attack aging itself. Piecemeal interventions can also cause problems because one pharmaceutical intervention might introduce a number of side effects. Often, this leads to doctors prescribing another medication to treat the side effects of the first medication, and treating a series of symptoms can lead to a cycle of overmedication. While the Orange perspective benefits from the great respect it affords science, it can be limited by not considering a more holistic approach.

Quadrant 4 – *Corporate/Governmental/Institutional Influences*

The Orange perspective highly values power, money, and personal advancement, and the companies, corporations, and business organizations that engage with this perspective are no exception. Applying the latest scientific research, they create products, weapons, medicines, and other technologies they can use or sell to become wealthier and more powerful. These corporations know that many of their customers also value science, so they may use scientific jargon and buzzwords in advertising some of their products, whether or not the claims are scientifically supported.

In addition, the Orange viewpoint, which tends not to be holistic, can benefit "Big Pharma" because it can be more lucrative to treat a bunch of different symptoms of aging rather than the root causes of aging itself. With this interest in profit, research funding focused on addressing the root causes of aging may be limited.

Governments that take an Orange perspective are more likely than those with a Blue view to support scientific research into health and wellness and fund programs designed to improve public health. For better or worse, this benefits drug corporations that profit from interventions that only treat disease symptoms. For Big Pharma, this has become the status quo. On the one hand, it serves the public by providing them with the latest medicines that manage disease symptoms. On the other hand, the public isn't really helped if a piecemeal approach to just managing symptoms is followed. Because of limited funding, research that focuses on alleviating a myriad of symptoms, not the root causes of aging, may prevail. This focus on simply treating symptoms promotes a culture of pill-popping seniors. In her later years, John's Mom took 13 pills daily, nearly half of which she took to address the side effects of others. Relying on medications to combat symptoms of aging can distract the aged from adopting fundamental lifestyle changes that are less expensive, less risky (fewer meds with serious side effects), healthier, and more sustainable (eating right and exercising).

An excellent example of this is type II diabetes. Interventions lean towards prescribing drugs rather than addressing root causes through lifestyle changes. Drug companies have made lots of money off drugs, taking advantage of people's tendency to take the easy way out by using pills, which further diminishes their motivation to adopt healthier lifestyle changes. Often, for companies and institutions to support healthy lifestyle changes, it must help their bottom line.

A case in point is the healthcare insurance industry, which has a vested financial interest in people keeping healthy for longer. The cost of covering catastrophic or chronic illnesses places a significant financial burden on these institutions. Conversely, healthy people generally rely less on medical interventions, and health insurance companies now recognize the financial benefits of healthy subscribers. As a result, many health insurance companies cover or subsidize the costs of subscriber behaviors that reflect healthy lifestyle choices (e.g., gym memberships, smoking cessation programs, annual physicals, and vaccinations).

WHY DOES IT MATTER?

When reading through these examples, you might have thought that the Orange perspective promotes anti-aging interventions better than Blue, which may be true in many cases. However, each of these perspectives, as well as the other six, offer their own benefits and drawbacks. There are several ways that people with a Blue view might support anti-aging interventions without betraying the worldview they value. Firstly, some religions and cultures support healthy lifestyles. Furthermore, those at the Blue level of development often value extended family as part of their purpose in life and consider it their primary responsibility to be there for their spouse, children, and grandchildren for as long as possible. They may also view life as sacred and a blessing, thus making them more likely to take steps to prolong it.

Overall, every Level of Development involves tendencies that could be beneficial or detrimental when it comes to health and embracing anti-aging interventions. For example, those within the Purple (Animistic-Magical) level are likely to respect their elders for the wisdom that comes with age and may be less fearful of growing old and being shunned (Quadrant 2 – "We" Space-Cultural). However, a strong belief that spiritual forces determine life outcomes can reduce a person's likelihood of embracing scientific advancements (Quadrant 3 – "It" Space-Behavioral). For a different example, under the Green (Sensitive Self) paradigm, empathy and understanding are the goals (Quadrant 2 – "We" Space-Cultural). People with this Green perspective will likely stand behind progressive social programs that promote public health education or access to medical treatment (Quadrant 4 – "Its" Space-Social). However, the value the Green view places on dialogue and consensus can be crippling to the advancement of anti-aging lifestyles if there is no unanimous agreement on the right way to proceed.

Many people across Levels of Development (with the exception of the "being levels") might not want to live longer lives even if they knew they could age reasonably healthy. They project that outliving family and friends would result in losing one's identity, not belonging, and being alone.

These examples show that a person's Level of Development plays a significant role in how they think about aging and anti-aging interventions. Therefore, it's essential to understand Levels of Development and their influence on how we process or interpret information from the four quadrants. By opening our minds and expanding our thinking beyond current limitations, we can embrace new ideas and technologies that can afford us longer and healthier lives.

It all starts with YOU.

To affect change in our lives, we must find a way to go beyond the paradigms ingrained in us to see aging from a more comprehensive perspective. In other words, we need to embrace a viewpoint that incorporates aspects from multiple Levels of Development, which is a viewpoint more reminiscent of the "being levels," Yellow (Integrative) or even Turquoise (Holistic). What is necessary for this more comprehensive perspective? We firmly believe it begins with the individual, who believes there is another, more holistic, and life-supporting way to live and extend life. To be that person, you must be willing to learn, take responsibility for your health, and make choices that promote longevity. To fully embrace an anti-aging lifestyle, one must stand firmly in the first quadrant (I-Space) and take charge. This takes courage. There is a vast difference between doing this and feeling like a victim of circumstance. Pointing the finger at someone or something else is the easy way out and is why many of us don't have what we want in life. If, as we will discuss later, aging is a disease in and of itself and can be cured, it challenges everything we have been taught. We may not be able to live forever (yet), but we can take steps to ensure that we age well. Help is available. Here are some tips to prepare you for your anti-aging journey, should you choose this adventure.

Objective Examination

It can be helpful to step back from your personally ingrained perspective and look at aging objectively. One of the ways you could do this is to write out as many of your beliefs on health, medicine, science, aging, and anti-aging interventions as you can think of, and then take a step back to look at them as an impartial observer. If it helps, you could imagine yourself as an anthropologist, journalist, or even a space alien trying to understand the belief system in front of you! Next, consider the pros and cons of the beliefs you've written down *concerning promoting longevity.* Are they helpful or limiting? What other perspectives would be more valuable? Do this while you're healthy and active—don't wait for a scare, such as a heart attack or stroke, to start thinking about these things.

Consider the Value in Life

Regardless of how you feel about death and how life outcomes are determined, try to see the value in life and longevity. Having a longer lifespan and health span allows you to spend more time with loved ones, enjoy your hobbies and passions, see more of the world, have memorable experiences, and achieve more in your career and other endeavors. A longer health span also allows you to take advantage of future advancements in improving longevity. A much longer and healthier life than you ever expected may be in your grasp if you start working on improving your physiology sooner rather than later.

Explore the Possibilities

Do you feel like there's nothing you can do about aging? Learning about advancements and discoveries in medical science can convince you this isn't true. Science is revealing more about the process of aging each and every day, and this will likely lead to new ways to treat it!

Resist the Status Quo

Remember that cultural forces and social groups also subscribe to one paradigm or another. They may not be supportive of your attempts to combat aging, or they may be suspicious of new scientific advancements. Don't be discouraged if your family and friends don't support you. They are just as influenced by their Levels of Development as anyone else. If your doctor seems committed to the piecemeal approach of medicating each age-related disease as it arises instead of helping you to change your lifestyle to prevent them, don't let this hold you back, either. Drug companies, too, have a vested interest in pushing this viewpoint, as they stand to profit from selling more medications, regardless of the adverse side effects they may present. Finally, remember that popular culture pushes against many healthy lifestyle changes and can overtly or insidiously push you to overeat (super-sized meals), over-drink (Big Gulp), and over-medicate (a pill for everything) to get you to spend more money. Sugar is added to virtually every packaged food for a reason— it's addictive and will keep you coming back even though it's unhealthy!

Don't Give Up

You are pushing against dozens or hundreds of societal forces, as well as many ingrained habits, as you seek to improve your lifestyle to combat the effects of aging. It may be challenging, especially at first! However, press on and be as persistent as you can. It won't always be so hard, either. Although a bit of a challenge initially, we found a new way of eating that expanded our palette and was quite enjoyable. If you want anti-aging medical support, a growing number of doctors specializing in "integrative medicine" are joining the field, so see if you can find one in your area! Finally, the anti-aging movement is growing, so you'll likely find like-minded people to share information and offer support locally or online. You can find our Facebook group "Anti-Aging Explorers" online, comprised of like-minded people interested in living long, healthy lives.

If you can lovingly hold yourself accountable, you can find ways to make an anti-aging lifestyle work.

We are about to present information about some fundamental shifts in how diseases of aging are defined and reveal several new approaches to advance anti-aging and longevity. But we can't emphasize enough how important it is to be open to the science behind recent breakthroughs in aging and be willing to consider lifestyle changes that can promote health and longevity. If you subscribe to the notion that there is nothing we can do about aging because it's simply a fact of life and your perspective is unlikely to change, then there is little value in reading on. Conversely, if you are willing to move around and across human Levels of Development and objectively process the information you seek and receive, you will be excited to read about the possibilities offered by the latest innovative anti-aging interventions.

In the next section, we will delve into the fascinating, cutting-edge science that considers aging as a disease in and of itself, as well as the latest interventions that can be applied to slow, treat, and even reverse the effects of aging.

THE IMPORTANCE OF GUIDANCE

"Aging is not 'lost youth' but a new stage of opportunity and strength."

— BETTY FRIEDAN

As you may recall from the introduction, our personal backgrounds played a huge role in writing this book. As soon as we began implementing our lifestyle changes, we felt the difference, and with our joint weight loss and John's improvement with his hip pain, we became devoted to sharing what we've learned with more people.

As a society, we've come to accept that getting older automatically equates to a decline in our health and a limitation on what we can do, both physically and mentally. But just as air and water quality have improved through a shift in how we operate globally, our health can improve when we make sustainable lifestyle changes.

This is such a daunting idea, though, and we've spoken to many people who say they know they need to improve their overall health but don't have a clue where to start. We want to simplify that process and believe this book is the answer.

With that in mind, we'd like to ask you a favor. You can help us to reach more people by taking just a few minutes to write a short review. People are always looking for clear and easy-to-follow guidance to help them understand and implement the changes they know they need to make, and reviews make it much easier for them to find what they're looking for.

By leaving a review of this book on Amazon, you'll shine a light on the guidance those readers are searching for, ultimately helping them to make the changes needed to improve their health and quality of life dramatically.

Simply by telling other readers how this book has helped you and what they'll find inside, you'll show them exactly where they can find the guidance they're looking for.

Thank you for your support. Aging doesn't have to mean a decline in health and well being... In fact, it shouldn't. Thank you for helping us in our mission to share the knowledge we know can make an incredible difference.

Scan the QR code below for a quick review!

PART III: JOINING THE REVOLUTION!

 "You can't help getting older, but you don't have to get old."

— GEORGE BURNS

Now that we have established the importance of reflecting on how we see the world and the topic of aging, let's introduce some novel, scientific ideas about aging. To begin with, the phrase "age-related diseases" is an interesting one. It describes a group of linked illnesses, disorders, and conditions because they include age as a risk factor. In other words, aging increases your risk of developing one of these conditions. Most people will encounter one or more of them as they grow older. Age-related diseases are still diagnosed and treated as separate issues— the long list of medications prescribed for older adults can attest to that. However, the latest scientific research suggests that we should look at aging as a disease in and of itself, with the current line-up of age-related diseases as symptoms. According to several sources, aging meets the criteria for "defining" a disease. For example, the Merriam-Webster dictionary defines disease as "a condition of the living animal or plant body or one of its parts that impairs normal functioning and is typically manifested by distinguishing signs and symptoms." The World Health Organization defines a disease as "any harmful deviation from the normal functional and structural state of the organism, generally associated with specific signs and symptoms and differing in nature from physical injury" (WHO, 2020). Aging is unique as a disease since it will inevitably affect all human beings who don't die from other causes (e.g., car accidents, plane crashes, or war).

Aging can make everyday life more problematic as it has well-known effects on the cells, tissues, and organs of the body. For example, bones become more brittle, muscle mass is lost, tissues become drier and less flexible, cognitive function declines, the heart pumps less blood, metabolism slows, and, eventually, the condition is terminal. Typically, bodily changes associated with aging are considered outside the norm when the level of functioning the individual has enjoyed since puberty is degraded.

If science suggests aging can be viewed as a disease in and of itself, why shouldn't we search for ways to treat it like we do for other diseases? Individuals operating under certain Levels of Development or paradigms may profess that, indeed, there is nothing we can do about aging. There is no way to hold off the march of time forever! While "forever" may be a stretch, the most cutting-edge scientific research suggests that the bodily changes that occur due to aging don't have to be inevitable or irreversible. Treating aging as a disease would allow us to tackle all of the symptoms of age-related diseases more comprehensively at a fundamental level. This holistic perspective changes the way we approach aging across all quadrants, allowing us to look for innovative solutions that tackle aging at its roots instead of playing whack-a-mole with its symptoms.

Most people want to strive for the greatest length and quality of life possible (of course, how "quality of life" is defined depends on your Level of Development and your way of viewing the world). Despite differences in perspective, few would argue that we shouldn't attempt to treat the disease of aging using all of the information systems represented by the quadrants, even if we can't eventually cure it. The medical field has already developed numerous ways of slowing the progress of certain diseases or improving the quality of the patient's life, even if the condition eventually becomes terminal. Examples include radiation therapy, bone marrow transplants, and gene therapy for cancer. In addition, drugs have been developed to slow the progression of diseases and mitigate their symptoms, like Alzheimer's disease, macular degeneration, and Parkinson's disease. These successes give us every reason to believe that aging can be treated at seemingly more fundamental levels, enabling us to slow down or even reverse aging while alleviating its symptoms. Consequently, this would not just increase the lifespan of individuals but also improve their quality of life (health span).

A paradigm shift from the traditional view of treating age-related diseases separately to a more holistic view would be incredibly radical in a culture that sees aging as an inevitable part of life. Not only would this completely alter how we look at aging and age-related diseases, but it would also open the door to research into interventions often stifled by controversy (such as stem cell research). This paradigm shift might even lead to a "domino effect" throughout science and medicine. Would the medical establishment shift to this view regarding other illnesses and disorders? What if most of them are basically age-related? For example, would treating diseases become something that occurred at the epigenetic level by attacking the cause of the condition instead of simply attempting to mitigate the symptoms?

While it's impossible to tell what changes this paradigm shift would have on our society, the concept of fighting aging as a disease is revolutionary in and of itself, which is why we named this chapter "Joining the Revolution!" In this chapter, we will explore aging as a disease and its effects on the body, ranging from discussions on the physical hallmarks of aging to the biomechanical processes behind them. Finally, we'll look into what interventions are *currently* known to combat aging and those on the horizon. But, to fully understand how the interventions work, you first need to understand a bit of the science of aging itself.

KNOW YOUR ENEMY: THE NINE HALLMARKS OF AGING

The hallmarks of aging that we are about to discuss are drawn from the paradigm-changing book *Lifespan* by Dr. David Sinclair, a professor of genetics at Harvard Medical School, Co-Director of Harvard's Paul F. Glenn Center for Biology of Aging Research and world leader in anti-aging research. Sinclair is a proponent of the notion that aging is something that science and medicine can combat, pointing out in his book that the average life expectancy of humans is getting longer and longer as we learn more about the body and how it works. In addition, advancements in the science of aging point to the tell-tale biological markers of aging, which Sinclair refers to as the "hallmarks of aging."

Dr. Sinclair does not believe that aging necessarily places an unsurpassable ceiling on how long we can extend our lifespan as science advances its understanding of how to treat the hallmarks of aging to prevent the onset of age-related problems. Common diseases of the past, such as tuberculosis, were considered regular parts of life in their heydays, so there's no reason to believe that aging itself is undefeatable! However, making lifestyle changes allows you to start combating the hallmarks of aging without waiting on new medical advances. We hope that by understanding the molecular genetic reasons behind aging and the things you can do to combat it, this inside view will inspire you to make positive lifestyle changes available to you now. Below, we've given an overview of these hallmarks and what you can do to address them!

Attrition of the Telomeres

The human DNA molecule is so long that it would be impossible to store in a single cell without being carefully wound and packaged. Protein bodies called *histones* package DNA around themselves to protect it. It's like wrapping a thread around a spool so it's stored compactly without tangling. DNA that is wound around histones wraps itself further into a thicker molecule called *chromatin*, which then gets packaged into chromosomes. Humans have 23 pairs of chromosomes in each cell, which comprises our entire genetic code. Just like a thread can be unwrapped neatly from a spool for use, sections of a DNA strand can be unwound from a histone to be transcribed or replicated.

Our cells must completely replicate their DNA before they can divide, creating new cells to allow us to grow, repair injuries, and replace dead cells. As a result, billions of cells divide every day in the human body. However, the DNA replication process isn't perfect; consequently, a few base pairs, or "letters" in the genetic code, are lost at the ends of the molecule every time replication occurs. Fortunately, the ends of chromosomes contain extraneous sections of DNA. These sacrificial sections, called *telomeres*, protect the integrity of the rest of the DNA. These telomeres are regions of repetitive, meaningless base pair sequences that bear the brunt of this wear and tear, keeping the code we need safe!

However, with enough replications, even the telomeres get critically worn down. As a result, the ends of the molecule become exposed, resulting in adverse, cell-wide consequences. DNA damage at its ends can lead to genomic instability or problems with the DNA molecule itself that prevent the cell from functioning correctly. One of the consequences of genomic instability due to telomere attrition is the buildup of zombie cells, also known as *senescent cells*, which we will discuss in more detail in the dedicated section below.

What Can We Do About It?

In his book, where he discusses the benefits of regular exercise for increasing the human lifespan, Dr. Sinclair cites a study on the effect of exercise on telomeres in human blood cells. Researchers collected blood samples from a variety of adults with different exercise habits in this study. They discovered that those who exercised regularly had longer telomeres than those in their age groups who did not. With a sample size of thousands, this was a striking correlation. Another study showed that people who performed moderate exercise (equivalent to a 30-minute jog five days a week) had significantly longer telomeres than those in their age groups who exercised less. In fact, their telomeres resembled those of people a full decade younger than themselves!

Sinclair explains these amazing finds with the concept that, like fasting or caloric restriction, exercise places "good stress" on the body, also known as *hormesis*. Hormesis via exercise increases the amount of energy our cells produce by raising levels of the molecule NADH/NAD+, which is essential in the energy production process. Hormesis via exercise can also activate several genes that help the cell weather adversity, and many of these can promote longevity—two of these genes code for the sirtuins SIRT1 and SIRT6. *Sirtuins* are essential molecules that remove acetyl tags from histones, allowing the genes they carry to be activated or deactivated. For this reason, they fall into the category of *epigenetic regulators.* SIRT1 and SIRT6 also work to repair telomeres and protect them from further degradation. Finally, exercise also helps promote sirtuin activity by raising cellular levels of NADH/NAD+, which sirtuins use to perform their epigenetic function. All of these molecules are part of a network of the products of longevity-associated genes, which Sinclair calls the "survival circuit."

Genomic Instability

The human genome interacts with countless *enzymes,* or protein machines, every day. These enzymes have several roles, from unwinding or "unzipping" the DNA helix to reading the encoded genes, copying them as mRNA (transcription), and then "translating" the mRNA code into proteins at the ribosomes. This process occurs innumerable times a day in every cell in your body whenever a new protein needs to be synthesized. However, if there's something wrong with the DNA molecule itself—say, if it's damaged or broken—your cells won't be able to make proteins correctly, if at all. This will interfere with a cell's ability to replicate itself. In addition, if proteins, like sirtuins, preferentially focus on DNA repair, they can be distracted from performing other critical functions in the cell, which can cause harm

In *Lifespan,* Sinclair describes an experiment where he and his colleagues induced aging in cells by deliberately damaging the

DNA of younger yeast cells. Then, based on the suggestion of a newcomer to the lab, they inserted a second copy of SIR2 (which codes for important sirtuins) into the genomes of the yeast cells before trying the induced aging experiment again. This time, the yeast cells lived much longer with the damaged DNA than before. After additional research, Sinclair and his team concluded that DNA damage distracts sirtuins from their other roles as they scramble to repair the DNA molecule. This preferential focus on DNA repair leads to other problems throughout the cell, including sterility—a clear sign of aging in yeast (Sinclair, 2019).

In other words, every cell can sense when its DNA is damaged and sends molecules such as sirtuins to do repairs. Over time, the damage builds up, preventing these proteins from performing their other essential functions. Sinclair clarifies that these proteins aren't necessarily overwhelmed by the DNA damage but that the damage happens frequently enough that they don't have time to handle their previous functions before returning to the nucleus to fix another problem. The yeast in Sinclair's experiment that received another copy of the SIR2 gene lived longer, as they could produce and activate more of these essential proteins (Sinclair, 2019).

So how do DNA molecules become too damaged for sirtuins to keep up, leading to the adverse health effects we associate with aging? Although the DNA molecule is sequestered away in the nucleus to keep it safe, it can still be damaged over time by the compounds to which it's exposed. For example, environmental toxins and radiation can damage DNA over time. As previously mentioned, the body's process for replicating DNA is not perfect, so again, "errors" in the process build up. Finally, cells produce molecules called *free radicals* as a consequence of metabolism, which are oxidized chemical species that can damage DNA. While free radicals are no longer believed to be a significant cause of aging, they do cause unwanted DNA molecule mutations.

What Can We Do About It?

As mentioned in the previous section, hormesis refers to stress that activates positive genes associated with survival in the cell, including those that code for sirtuins. Fasting and exercise are both forms of hormesis that promote the activity of these genes in the cell—a process Sinclair calls the *survival circuit*. One could also boost the activity of sirtuins by raising the cell's levels of NAD+, which is required not only for mitochondrial function but for sirtuins to function correctly. Exercise can increase cellular levels of NAD+, but supplements that activate NAD+ are available on the market (see the supplement section at the end of this chapter).

Finally, reducing the amount of DNA damage that occurs in the first place can be helpful. You can reduce your contact with factors that contribute to DNA damage by wearing proper personal protective equipment (PPE) if working with potentially harmful chemicals and wearing sunscreen outdoors to protect yourself from the sun's radiation. Smoking is also a significant cause of DNA damage, so quitting should be a priority for any smoker seeking an anti-aging lifestyle.

Alterations to the Epigenome

Every cell in an organism has a copy of the entire genome. However, not all of the genome is active at the same time. Depending on a number of environmental and lifestyle factors, different genes are read and transcribed at various stages throughout your life to different degrees. At the same time, other genes are being "turned off" and not expressed. The epigenome controls the dynamic expression and suppression of genes throughout the body.

If this seems confusing, Sinclair provides the following helpful metaphor in *Lifespan*: If your body were a computer, your genetic code would be the hard drive, and your epigenome would be the installed software. Every computer is technically capable of performing any of the actions its processing power and hardware allow, but the quality of the software determines how well the computer actually functions. For example, if the software contains glitches or "bugs" or is corrupted by a virus, the computer cannot function properly. This computer analogy roughly illustrates how environmental factors and lifestyle choices can affect your epigenome and, therefore, how well your body functions. That is, poor lifestyle choices and adverse environmental exposures can have negative consequences regarding how well a person ages. Conversely, healthy lifestyle choices and environmental conditions can positively affect how one ages.

Examining how the epigenome affects aging requires us to understand the activity of sirtuins, which we discussed at length in previous sections. As we know, sirtuins have several jobs throughout the cell, one of which is to assist with storing human DNA around histones. Which genes are expressed depends heavily on which sections of the code are exposed. Sirtuin genes that expose sections of the code (*euchromatin*) allow it to be transcribed. On the other hand, sirtuin genes that keep code tightly wrapped around histones (*heterochromatin*) prevent transcriptions. Sirtuins play a critical role in controlling this by removing acetyl tags from histones, which designates that section of DNA as heterochromatin and prevents it from being transcribed.

Sinclair introduces a concept called *epigenetic noise*, which he likens to mistakes a pianist makes when playing a composition. Since nothing about a biological organism works properly every time, sometimes there are mistakes in the epigenome. When these are rare, the organism can continue to function normally. However, epigenetic noise can increase to a level that becomes overwhelming. For example, if a pianist plays a ton of notes besides those contained in the sheet music, the piece she's playing becomes unrecognizable. Similarly, once epigenetic noise increases to a certain point, it causes noticeable problems in the epigenome. Sinclair suggests that this phenomenon is responsible for many common symptoms of aging. For example, this could include the graying of hair, wrinkling of the skin, joint problems, and the ex-differentiation of cells. Ex-differentiation of cells occurs when the wrong genes are activated, resulting in changes to cells that cause them to behave in ways not originally intended.

So, where are these extra notes coming from in the piano analogy? When sirtuins are busy repairing DNA damage, they can't interact effectively with histones as epigenetic regulators, leading to random alterations in gene expression (like the random notes in the piano analogy). Sinclair describes this randomness as a "loss of information" and an "ultimate" cause of aging that forms the basis of his research.

What Can We Do About It?

Hormesis, once again, is essential here since activating sirtuins and other genes associated with longevity can fight against epigenetic noise by stabilizing the genome. The three best ways to promote hormesis are fasting, caloric restriction, and exercise. As stated above, exercise boosts sirtuin activity and raises cellular levels of NAD+. Sirtuins need NAD+ to function correctly as epigenetic regulators, which is essential to preventing epigenetic noise. Certain supplements can also help increase NAD+, activate sirtuins, and thus stabilize the genome.

DNA damage can also lead to alterations to the epigenome, resulting in genomic instability. Some ways to minimize DNA damage include avoiding harmful chemicals, heavy metals, or radiation, wearing sunscreen, and not smoking.

Loss of Proteostasis

The cellular pathways the body uses to produce proteins are very complex—that's why universities dedicate whole curriculums to this topic. But don't worry; we're just going to hit some of the basics. To begin with, the process that produces proteins is called *proteostasis*. This term comes from the word *homeostasis*, the "normal" self-regulated balance internally maintained by living organisms. If something goes wrong with the protein-making process, the proteins at work in the cell can become unstable and fail to perform their proper functions. Unstable proteins involved in the transcription and translation processes could lead to unwanted alterations in the epigenome and other impairments throughout the cell.

Along with ribosomes and the protein translation machinery, other compounds are involved in maintaining proteostasis in the cell. *Protein chaperones* are compounds that ensure that, when proteins are made, they fold into the correct shapes and stay there. *Ubiquitins* are molecules attached to a faulty protein to tag it for transport to a lysosome, where it is broken down and recycled. Proteostasis cannot be maintained if genomic instability, epigenomic alterations, or environmental toxins adversely affect protein chaperones and ubiquitins. Consequently, faulty unfolded and untagged proteins can accumulate in the cell's cytoplasm, adversely affecting the proteins around them. Accordingly, misfolded proteins can form, which then clump or aggregate together. These aggregates also damage the cell itself and make it harder for other proteins to work correctly, somewhat analogous to "one bad apple can spoil the whole bunch." Is the disruption of proteostasis really that important to health, wellness, and aging? It's thought that a loss of proteostasis is heavily involved in the development of age-related neurodegenerative diseases such as Alzheimer's and Parkinson's diseases (Lopez-Otin et al., 2013).

What Can We Do About It?

There's currently less information available about how to combat loss of proteostasis than other hallmarks of aging, but that doesn't mean there's nothing we can do. Since the loss of proteostasis is linked to genomic instability and alterations to the epigenome, combating these two hallmarks of aging are great ways to help maintain proteostasis.

Further, it has been shown that the loss of proteostasis and the formation of protein aggregates are associated with neurodegenerative diseases. Therefore, research into preventing these diseases might be worth investing in. Particularly, research into addressing obesity and related issues like diabetes might be relevant since these conditions are associated with the development of Alzheimer's and dementia (Alford et al., 2018), as is chronically poor sleep quality (Delic, Ratliff, and Citron, 2021).

Deregulated Nutrient Sensing

Hormones are one of the body's methods for signaling between cells and different organ systems. They are secreted from different types of cells throughout the body and travel through the bloodstream to be received by the receptors of other types of cells, thus transmitting a message. Hormones are most commonly thought of when it comes to their role in regulating puberty and menopause. However, hormones are involved in almost any biological process you can think of, from the stress response, regulating metabolism, to sensing the availability of nutrients in the body leading to feelings of hunger or satiety. Hormones can also trigger or block the secretion of other hormones. For example, *leptin*, which is associated with satiety, prevents the secretion of *ghrelin*, which is one of the hormones responsible for the feeling of hunger.

As we discussed above, one significant role of hormones is nutrient sensing. Our bodies are complex systems that require a lot of energy to function. This energy comes from food nutrients like carbohydrates, protein, and fat. When consumed, nutrients flow through the bloodstream, triggering the secretion of hormones that facilitate the uptake of the nutrients into cells and their conversion to energy. For example, insulin, secreted from the beta cells of the pancreas, facilitates glucose uptake when detected in the bloodstream. Hormones also stimulate extra energy storage, such as glycogen in the muscles and liver and fat in the adipose cells.

As mentioned above, insulin is secreted in response to rising blood sugar levels. However, the human body can become "deaf" to insulin. If the bloodstream has been dealing with high sugar levels, the body can start building up insulin resistance, just as it would to alcohol or another drug. Insulin resistance forces the pancreas to create more insulin to manage blood sugar, leading to a cycle that causes more and more resistance. Insulin resistance is a major warning sign for type II diabetes, a common and harmful age-related disease. Older people are much more at risk for type II diabetes as they age; however, it is being diagnosed in younger and younger individuals due to the modern prevalence of obesity.

Another critical player in the body's nutrient-sensing system is the complex of proteins encoded by the gene *TOR* (*mTOR* when found in mammals). The proteins encoded by mTOR are involved in your body's response to stress, including good stress, such as exercise and fasting. mTOR dictates how much protein your cells can make based on the number of available amino acids (base components of proteins). It pushes for growth when plenty is available. However, when amino acids are scarce, inhibition of mTOR will partially inhibit cell division while inducing cells to recycle waste material and other components in a renewing process called *autophagy*. Autophagy declines in aging individuals, leading to a buildup of harmful molecules in cells that can eventually inhibit their function.

What Can We Do About It?

While age is a risk factor for deregulated nutrient sensing, so are lifestyle choices. Eating a diet high in sugar, especially refined sugar, and being sedentary are two of the worst things you can do for your body's sensitivity to insulin and other forms of nutrient sensing. To combat insulin resistance, lifestyle changes are your best friends—regular exercise, a low-carb diet, and alternative eating plans such as caloric restriction and intermittent fasting.

Sinclair also cautions against overeating meat, especially red meat, when trying to combat aging with lifestyle changes. It's true that we need protein to survive and that meat contains all the amino acids needed to form proteins. However, it is possible to have *too much* of some essential amino acids.

Metformin is a medication commonly used to treat type II diabetes, but it is also growing in prominence as an anti-aging measure. People who medicate with Metformin for their blood sugar have been observed becoming healthier in other aspects of their lives. Several studies on mice indicated Metformin could potentially increase lifespan or health span. For example, one study showed that mice given a low dose of Metformin lived 6% longer than the control group. In addition, a survey of 68,000 people using Metformin to treat diabetes showed that the medication also seems to confer some protection against cancers, depression, dementia, and frailty (Sinclair, 2019).

Mitochondrial Dysfunction

You've probably heard the phrase "the mitochondria are the powerhouses of the cell," commonly used in high-school-level biology courses and brief explanations of metabolism in the media. *Mitochondria* are organelles (structures) found in almost all animal cells, and the biochemical reactions required to convert nutrients to energy occur in their matrixes and membranes. They have unique but smaller genomes and are strongly reminiscent of *prokaryotic cells* (simple cells that existed before plants and animals). Scientists believe their presence in animal and plant cells results from a symbiotic relationship between two types of organisms billions of years ago. While cell diagrams found in high school and even university textbooks generally depict cells with one mitochondrion, there are, in fact, many in each cell to produce all the energy that a cell needs to function.

So, what do the mitochondria have to do with aging? The number of mitochondria in a person's cells declines as they age, contributing to the lower energy levels experienced by many older individuals. Cellular levels of NAD+ decline as a person gets older. Previously, we discussed how low levels of NAD+ impair the function of sirtuins that act on a cell's nucleus. Similarly, lack of NAD+ impairs sirtuin activity in the mitochondria, resulting in less mitochondria replication and energy production.

Finally, as stated, mitochondria have their own genomes, which can mutate just as nuclear DNA can, and this mutation impairs mitochondrial function. Such mutations may occur due to increased levels of free radicals inside mitochondria, as these organelles produce more free radicals during metabolism as a person ages. However, Sinclair is doubtful that mutations caused by free radicals in mitochondrial DNA are a major cause of aging due to a significant amount of evidence to the contrary (Perez et al., 2009).

Mitochondrial dysfunction can lead to serious consequences as it progresses, such as impairment of organ function or even organ failure if an organ can no longer produce the energy it needs to keep working.

What Can We Do About It?

Undergoing hormesis of any kind is the best way to fight mitochondrial dysfunction. Whether intense exercise, caloric restriction, or intermittent fasting, hormesis pushes the survival-associated genes in the human genome into action, promoting health and longevity. Hormesis is known to boost NAD+, an essential molecule for energy production, but it also triggers the activation of a gene called AMPK. AMPK is responsible for restoring mitochondrial function when energy is in short supply. Exercise, especially strength and resistance training, causes cells to create more mitochondria over time to produce the energy required for the work. In addition, exercise raises cellular levels of NAD+. Caloric restriction is also shown to boost levels of alpha-ketoglutarate, which is used as a fuel by our mitochondria and can improve mitochondrial health. Alpha-ketoglutarate has been shown to extend the lifespan of nematode worms in a laboratory trial (Sinclair, 2019).

Accumulation of Senescent Cells

We already know that cells with damaged DNA could become cancerous if allowed to proliferate, but what mechanisms does the body have to combat this? Cells can enter a state called *senescence*, permanently removed from the cell lifecycle, and can no longer grow and divide. Senescent cells have been referred to as "zombie cells" by several sources, as they are still *technically* alive but are no longer fulfilling their original function. Instead, senescent cells secrete harmful compounds, including inflammatory mediators, that adversely affect cells around them. Unfortunately, these destructive cells build up as we age. So how does this happen?

Recall that *telomeres*, the caps at the end of our DNA molecules that prevent the strand from fraying, wear down with each replication and limit how many times a cell can divide. The upper limit is 40-60 divisions, known as the Hayflick Limit, named after the scientist who discovered it. As you'll see in the *Exhaustion of Stem Cells* section below, the stem cells of our bodies are special in many ways, one of them being the presence of the enzyme *telomerase,* which repairs telomeres, allowing an older stem cell to keep replicating without mutations. However, "mistakes," damage, or other alterations in DNA sequences (see *Genomic Instability* and *Alterations to the Genome)* that appear over time could cause cells to multiply out of control. This out-of-control replication could lead to cancer. Fortunately, the gene for telomerase is inactive in the non-stem cells throughout our bodies to limit how many times a cell can divide and, therefore, the likelihood that cancer will manifest.

Our cells have a signaling system that triggers a cellular response when the DNA molecule is broken and an exposed end of a DNA strand is detected. A short telomere tends to lose its protective histone packaging, exposing the end of its DNA strand and triggering a damage response by the cell. The DNA repair response includes proteins known as sirtuins that rush to the rescue. In a normal situation, this repair effort would connect or ligate two broken pieces of DNA. However, in the case of a critically short telomere, these efforts do more harm than good, connecting different chromosomes together and massively altering the DNA sequence. As a result, the cell can no longer replicate its DNA to divide and behaves erratically.

When the senescent cell's signaling system perceives something is wrong but cannot fix the problem, it alerts nearby cells of danger. It sends out panic signals in the form of *cytokines,* which trigger the same inflammatory response from healthy cells nearby. This response summons *macrophages,* a common type of immune cell, to the scene. Besides mediating the inflammatory response, macrophages are responsible for eating and digesting infected or damaged cells and invaders like foreign bacteria. As no foreign threat is present, the macrophages start to attack healthy tissue, leading to tissue damage over time and chronic inflammation. To make matters worse, the "panic" signal secreted by senescent cells can also cause other cells to become senescent, hence the "zombie" moniker. Cancers in older people may be linked to this process.

What Can We Do About It?

The main problem created by senescent cells is the chronic inflammation they cause. Lifestyle choices that reduce inflammation throughout the body can be one way to combat this hallmark. These include: cutting out inflammatory foods like processed and cured meats, pre-packaged snacks, and refined sugars, taking certain supplements, eating healthier, and considering an alternative eating plan like intermittent fasting.

Exhaustion of Stem Cells

Stem cell research is a hot topic, but many people are unfamiliar with stem cells and their massive potential for combating the hallmarks of aging. Stem cells are "undifferentiated" cells that are pushed down different differentiation pathways as they multiply, developing into each type of cell we see in the human body. Epigenetics is responsible for determining which types of cells the body needs. In the epigenome, intercellular signaling molecules help determine a stem cell's fate (i.e., kidney or muscle cell). Eventually, a differentiating stem cell will "commit" to a particular cell lineage. There's a point of no return where the genes that would allow that cell to change to another kind are turned off, also driven by epigenetics. On the other hand, some stem cells don't differentiate and instead continuously divide to keep a healthy population of stem cells in the body.

There are different kinds of stem cells, and the difference matters. *Embryonic* stem cells found in fertilized ova three to five days old are known as *blastocysts,* one of the earliest stages of fetal development in mammals. These stem cells rapidly divide and can still develop into any other kind of cell. As the fetus develops, is born, and then grows up, the prevalence of stem cells decreases, but adults still have stem cell reserves in the bone marrow, fat, and other select locations throughout the body. Stem cells found in adults are restricted in what kind of cells they can become. They are useful to the body for replenishing specific populations of cells that die off and can't reproduce themselves through mitosis, such as white blood cells that fight disease. The body also uses stem cells to facilitate growth and repair damage.

Unfortunately, one characteristic of aging is that stem cells become "exhausted" over time, making it harder to repair injuries or fight off diseases. Stem cells lose their ability to divide as we age due to epigenetic noise, genomic instability, or cells becoming senescent. If stem cells cannot replenish themselves, the rest of the body suffers the consequences, just like how knocking over one domino will cause those behind it to fall as well. For example, stem cell exhaustion leads to a decline in the immune system. This decline explains why infectious diseases are often more dangerous to older adults—as they are less able to replenish the white blood cells that fight infection.

What Can We Do About It?

Currently, stem cell therapies can replace stem cells. These therapies are medical interventions that transplant or infuse stem cells into a person's body. The body can use these supplemental stem cells to replenish declining cell populations. For example, the immune system declines as people age, and new stem cells can differentiate to boost declining populations of immune cells and help fight off infections. The most common form of stem cell therapy is a bone marrow transplant. These procedures have helped treat cancer and slow the progress of neurodegenerative, age-related diseases like Alzheimer's and Parkinson's. In addition, stem cell therapy has helped with vision loss and arthritic joints. Much of the physical decline associated with aging is linked to stem cell exhaustion, and while stem cell therapy is not accessible to everyone, it is growing in popularity. It may become part of more people's anti-aging toolboxes as scientific understanding of the benefits increases.

Altered Intercellular Communication

Scientists are learning more and more about how the systems that make up our bodies really are inherently interconnected. For example, cells regularly communicate not just with their direct neighbors but with other cells located near and far throughout the body. They do this by secreting a range of molecules that travel through the bloodstream or the extracellular space, connecting to protein receptors on the surface of other cells. These molecules trigger a reaction in the cell receiving the signal. Cells secrete signaling molecules for a vast range of purposes. Examples of why signals are sent include warning other cells about danger, triggering apoptosis (programmed death) in faulty cells, prompting a cell to move toward the source of the signal (chemotaxis), and causing the secretion of another signaling molecule. A major class of protein signaling molecules is called *cytokines*, many of which have inflammatory properties.

So what makes altered intercellular communication a hallmark of aging? The short answer is that altered intercellular communication contributes to chronic inflammation, which, in turn, promotes aging. Inflammation is a common immune reaction that relies on intercellular signaling to function. The purpose of inflammation is to make a part of the body inhospitable to invaders by increasing the temperature and blood flow to bring in immune cells, such as macrophages, which secrete additional inflammatory factors and physically attack the threat. Macrophages engage in *phagocytosis*, where invaders such as bacteria and foreign materials are "eaten" by the cell and digested. It's perfectly normal to experience inflammation when an actual threat is present. For example, if you've ever had a cut or scratch grow hot, red, and swollen, the injury is inflamed to combat bacteria that might otherwise have entered your body. In a healthy person, this inflammation decreases once the threat gets resolved.

However, many people are dealing with chronic inflammation throughout the body when no foreign invader is present. Chronic inflammation can be linked to obesity, diet, and other factors that affect our epigenetics. In addition, inflammation is involved in almost every age-related disease, from heart disease to diabetes to neurodegenerative conditions. While short-term inflammation is an important defense mechanism, chronic inflammation can damage cells and tissues. This inflammation can be a red flag for several health problems, many related to age. Chronic inflammation is linked to heart disease and associated conditions, including *atherosclerosis*. In atherosclerosis, cholesterol plaques build up in the arteries, which then become inflamed, summoning macrophages to attack the plaques. This response leads to the hardening of the arterial wall and a narrowing of the space inside the blood vessel, a serious risk factor for heart attacks and other forms of heart disease. In many cases, a chronic inflammatory response is symptomatic of how epigenetic damage, resulting from an unhealthy lifestyle and environmental threats, can alter intercellular communication.

Altered intercellular communication can also arise due to malfunctioning cells, and chronic inflammation is a prime example. Recall that senescent cells secrete numerous inflammatory signaling molecules, which call the cells around them to "panic" and become senescent as well, secreting more and more inflammatory molecules. Chronic inflammation is so heavily linked to aging that scientists have even coined the term "inflammaging" to describe inflammation's pervasive role in aging. For example, inflammation activates a molecule called Nf kappaB (NF-KB) in cells, which is a factor in how cells respond to inflammatory signals. When NF-KB is active in a hypothalamus's cells for an extended period, these cells reduce the amount of gonadotropin-releasing hormone (GnRH) they secrete. Reduced levels of GnRH lead to several negative consequences of aging, such as bone and muscle weakness, as well as reducing the formation of new brain connections (neurogenesis). It has been shown that restoring GnRH to the aging brain can reverse the loss of neurogenesis (Zhang et al., 2013).

What Can We Do About It?

Reducing inflammation is one of the most important aspects of countering aging through lifestyle changes. Healthy lifestyles will help prevent and negate the effects of inflammatory molecules secreted from senescent or damaged cells, reducing your risk of developing age-related diseases associated with chronic inflammation. Diet is one of the most important factors in reducing inflammation. Many foods are linked to high levels of inflammation throughout the body, including red meat, packaged snacks, high-sodium foods, processed meats, and refined carbohydrates or sugars. Another part of your diet that may contribute to chronic inflammation is lectins, including wheat germ agglutinin (WGA). Lectins are proteins found in plants that are harmful to your digestive system. Lectins bind to carbohydrates, including carbohydrates on the surface of cells. When this happens with cells lining the digestive tract, it can cause inflammation, damage the integrity of the gut lining, interfere with nutrient absorption, and harm your gut microbiome. WGA is a common lectin found in wheat and a very potent initiator of inflammation in the gut.

Along with wheat, other foods with high lectin content include other grains, peanuts, raw legumes, raw soybeans, and raw potatoes. You can often reduce a food's lectin content by cooking it thoroughly. Bottom line, inflammation can be controlled by reducing the amount of lectins in our diet.

Finally, sirtuins, which, as discussed in previous sections, are activated by hormesis, can also work to reduce inflammation. Sirtuin activity can be boosted by triggering hormesis through fasting, caloric restriction, or exercise, as well as taking supplements that imitate the effects of these activities.

In addition to these "9 Hallmarks of Aging," one crucial macro system within the body most susceptible to poor lifestyle choices is our intestinal tract, or "gut." Poor gut health can directly contribute to aging. A healthy gut microbiome is essential for everyone, not just those concerned with aging and longevity. Did you know that gut bacteria can communicate with mitochondria in your cells? The following section will discuss why caring for our gut is so important.

THE IMPORTANCE OF THE GUT MICROBIOME

> *"The road to health is paved with good intestines!"*
>
> — SHERRY A. ROGERS

A healthy person's intestines contain billions of microorganisms from thousands of species, and the relationships between the human body and these microorganisms are just as diverse. These diverse relationships range from symbiotic (where both the human body and the bacteria benefit from the relationship) to commensal (where the bacteria benefit from living inside the body, but the body is not positively or negatively affected) to actively harmful (where damaging bacterial species contribute to disease in the human body).

Helpful bacteria are essential to the body's health in several ways. First and foremost, gut bacteria are necessary for proper digestion. They break down long-chain carbohydrates that we cannot digest ourselves, producing metabolites we can use. Of course, they do not do this to be nice. These bacteria break down and metabolize fiber to provide energy for themselves, with the helpful metabolites they produce being a pleasant side effect for us! Breaking down fiber makes it ready to be fermented in the gut, producing short-chain fatty acids (SCFAs) metabolized for energy by the cells of the large intestine's endothelial layer.

Consequently, these cells thrive, strengthening the gut wall, which keeps the nutrient absorption process running smoothly. Vitamins are also among the helpful metabolites produced by gut bacteria, especially B vitamins. Riboflavin, folate, and vitamin B12, for example, are all produced by lactic acid bacteria, a group of bacterial species that make their homes in our guts.

Gut bacteria also help defend us from infections by "crowding out" pathogens in the gut. Some places along the intestinal lining are better than others regarding access to space and nutrition. Resident bacteria compete with foreign invaders to occupy these spaces, keeping unwanted pathogens from gaining a foothold. In addition, some bacterial species produce metabolites that help the immune system fight or attack invaders directly.

We mentioned above that not all gut bacteria are helpful. When the population of gut bacteria becomes less diverse, colonies of harmful species can proliferate and contribute to illness and disease. Many maladies are linked to poor digestion or issues with the digestive tract, such as irritable bowel syndrome and inflammatory bowel disease. Previously, gut health had been considered unrelated to many aging-related illnesses. Recent science suggests otherwise. For example, Alzheimer's disease, heart disease, and diabetes are related to poor gut health (Gundry, 2019).

Some bacteria can make their homes inside tumors, protecting them from anti-cancer drugs. Thanks to this discovery, many cancer patients now undergo genomic testing to identify these bacteria and determine which antibiotics can best target them (Sinclair, 2019).

With each new study released, we are still learning more about the wide-reaching effects of the gut microbiome. For example, gut bacteria help modulate the immune system (Goldman, 2016). In addition, they can also affect mental health, as harmful gut bacteria can contribute to anxiety and depression (Gundry, 2019).

In the next section, we will look at how to apply our current knowledge of the causes of aging to combat these causes. You don't have to wait for new medical advancements to make anti-aging interventions. Instead, by adopting scientifically supported lifestyle changes today, you can start slowing the progress of aging in your own body right now.

HOW TO START FIGHTING

We've already touched on how to combat aging in your daily life, but how does this become a cohesive plan? A significant part of fighting aging is through lifestyle changes that support a healthy genome. Many of the hallmarks of aging are associated with inflammation (inflammaging), an example being senescent cells secreting inflammatory molecules. One way to counteract this is to eat in a manner that does not promote inflammation. For example, cutting out certain foods, like those containing lectins, can help reduce inflammation in the digestive tract. In addition, extensive studies have shown that caloric restriction can significantly lower inflammatory biomarkers (Meydani SN et al.).

Furthermore, a supplement regimen can provide your body with the tools it needs to counteract the hallmarks of aging. Supplements can serve a wide range of purposes, depending on what you're taking. For example, some supplements support the health of your gut microbiome, and others replace proteins or other factors that decline as you age. Still, others combat the effects of harmful dietary ingredients like lectins and sugar, to name just a few examples! Hopefully, we've made the biological or "inside" view of aging vivid enough that you've gained a greater appreciation for how deeply your body is affected by what you consume.

Re-Engineering Your Diet

 "Let food be thy medicine and medicine be thy food."

— HIPPOCRATES

There's a common saying that weight loss takes place in the kitchen. This adage can also apply to most, if not all, healthy lifestyle changes, including anti-aging interventions. However, even if you take supplements, find a healthy community, and exercise regularly, you won't reap the full benefit of these lifestyle changes if you're still eating a diet high in refined carbohydrates, red meat, processed snacks, and saturated fat! This section concerns modifications you might consider making to your diet to extend your lifespan and health span, as well as the science behind them.

Keeping in mind the four quadrants of human existence, we can see how each quadrant influences what we eat. For example, it's already well-established that certain foods increase chronic inflammation, and the current scientific data supports and expands upon that understanding (Quadrant 3 – Scientific/Technological Influences). Therefore, it makes sense for society to put this knowledge into practice (Quadrant 4 – Corporate/Governmental/Institutional influences), but this kind of change starts with the individual (Quadrant 1 – Personal Beliefs/Understandings/Experiences).

Currently, large corporations that control our drug and food production, sometimes known as Big Pharma and Big Ag, have yet to fully embrace the latest science regarding preventive medicine and healthy eating, as they are driven in other directions by profit. Researching and producing more nutritious, less processed foods is challenging and less profitable. If people practiced a healthier lifestyle because all quadrants supported it, think of all the existing medicines and treatments that would become obsolete and foods that would fall by the wayside! Big Pharma does provide treatments for some of the symptoms of aging, but many of these come with unwanted side effects or adverse long-term consequences. In the case of Big Ag, they're currently deriving a lot of profit from selling low-quality, addictive foods in greater and greater quantities. Therefore, we must take matters into our own hands to get our anti-aging health routines off the ground and have the fortitude to persist while waiting for the rest of society and culture to catch up. This doesn't mean you have to go it alone. You can find like-minded people to get support (check out our "Anti-Aging Explorers" group on Facebook).

Taking on a new diet can be very eye-opening. As we conducted research for this book and reflected on how heavily we are all influenced by corporate marketing efforts, we were amazed at how much this impacts our day-to-day lives. For example, if you're on a road trip, good luck finding a fast-food restaurant that serves healthy food. You have to take personal responsibility and plan ahead because your options are institutionally limited. Next time you go to the grocery store, notice how only a few aisles are labeled something along the lines of "health food" or "natural food." Ironically, many of these products are neither healthy nor natural! For example, foods marketed as gluten-free can be high in sugar, simple carbohydrates, or unhealthy fats (not to mention lectins). In addition, in the health food section you'll find gluten- or dairy-free versions of packaged foods, like cookies, which are packed with sugar and sold at higher prices than their regular counterparts. Knowing about and finding truly healthy foods takes more time and effort. We have had to up our game when it comes to reading labels, and thank goodness foods are required to have labels so consumers can be informed. Full disclosure—we've been duped occasionally with some foods we've purchased because we didn't read the ingredients label closely enough.

Also, it's common that healthy foods often cost more (e.g., organic vegetables, gluten-free pretzels, coconut milk, etc.) Still, we have decided the extra cost is worth it to practice a healthy lifestyle that promotes longevity. Also, we anticipate savings in medical bills, medicines, etc., which will offset the additional cost of buying healthy groceries! In addition, the cost of purchasing organic fruits and vegetables, though expensive now, may come down as more and more people buy them. In other words, as organic fruits and vegetables become popular, organic farming will grow as well, and hopefully, this increase in production will reduce costs.

Regarding the thoughts above on Quadrants 1, 3, and 4 and their influences, Quadrant 2 (family/community/cultural influences) is just as important because it can positively or negatively influence us. We have found this anti-aging journey easier because we have embarked upon it together. Not to say that it hasn't been fun, but together it's become a lifestyle. We've had a great time discovering the benefits of calorie restriction and intermittent fasting and exploring new healthy foods that are just as tasty and satisfying as those we gave up. And finally, we discovered supplements that specifically help combat many of the nine hallmarks of aging. Again, working together has made all the difference.

In the following section, we'll get into the benefits of calorie restriction and intermittent fasting, which are often not popular because they are perceived as difficult. Still, we wanted to discuss them first because they are so powerful in stimulating certain anti-aging biological processes.

Caloric Restriction and Intermittent Fasting

In modern Western society, most of us are used to grazing or snacking throughout the day. Many people can have a processed snack in their hands almost as soon as a craving strikes them. Next time you're out and about, take note of all the avenues for people to get their hands on unhealthy food on a whim. Between fast food restaurants, vending machines, food trucks, grocery aisles lined with packaged treats, and candy displays at check-out counters, you might lose track of all the opportunities to eat junk by the end of the day! Many people also experience anxiety around being hungry, which causes them to balk at cutting snacks from their diet. Shrewd marketing campaigns from snack companies have capitalized on the idea of constantly eating. Such suggestive corporate marketing is an excellent example of the potential negative impact of Quadrant 4 (corporate and governmental influences)!

However, this way of eating isn't natural or healthy. Our ancient ancestors likely ate much less than we do today—either in the form of fewer calories overall or going longer stretches between meals—and they didn't starve to death while doing it! Fasting and caloric restriction are good examples of hormesis or good stress, which activate longevity genes, induce autophagy's renewing process, and promote weight loss with all its other health benefits.

As an aside, some medications, such as Metformin (a drug used to manage blood sugar levels) or supplements like NAD+ boosters and EGCG, activate the same genes that fasting does— effectively creating a fasting-like state while you're still eating! Sinclair calls these genes the *survival circuit*, as they all help the cell weather stressful situations while promoting longevity.

Sinclair also notes that the benefits of fasting or caloric restriction aren't an excuse to eat *too little*, which is very dangerous. It's possible to become underweight or malnourished by restricting food to an unreasonable extent. However, healthily restricting food, either by intermittent fasting (forgoing food entirely for a set period) or caloric restriction (eating a smaller amount than usual), can do wonders for your health in numerous ways.

In conclusion, to quote the book *Lifespan*: "After 25 years of researching aging and having read thousands of scientific papers, if there is one piece of advice I can offer, one surefire way to stay healthy longer, one thing you can do to maximize your lifespan right now, it's this: eat less" (Sinclair, 2019).

What Is Caloric Restriction (CR)?

Simply put, caloric restriction is the practice of eating less food, either ongoingly or for a specific amount of time. This does not mean consistently eating less food than you need or denying your body the nutrition it needs to function. Again, starvation and malnutrition can have serious health consequences, including organ damage and death. However, ample evidence shows that reducing calories while maintaining adequate nutrition can still place cells under hormesis, activating the genes that promote survival and longevity.

Sinclair references a couple of dozen CR studies on mice, demonstrating that limiting calories without starvation or malnutrition lengthens lifespan. From these results, he feels the best action would be to eat only what your body *needs* to function and no more (Sinclair, 2019). But, unfortunately, it's difficult for most people, especially in the Western culture, to tolerate hunger for an extended period, i.e., long enough to record results about whether or not CR lengthens human lives.

Ken Wilbur suggests the frameworks of Quadrant 2 (family/community/cultural influences) and Quadrant 4 (corporate, governmental, and institutional influences) show that humans are deeply influenced by the people around them and the support systems in which they live. This suggests that positive influences from these Quadrants could reduce the quantity of food people eat and show that CR works for humans.

Here is a case in point: The island of Okinawa, part of Japan, is known for its unusually high population of centenarians and is considered a *Blue Zone*. The term Blue Zone was coined by Dan Buettner, author of *The Blue Zones*, a book investigating the cultures and lifestyles of the longest-lived people in the world. Sinclair references a study indicating that Okinawan school-children take in 25% fewer calories than their counterparts in the rest of Japan, while Okinawan adults consume 20% fewer calories than other Japanese adults. To sum it up, the Okinawan culture naturally supports CR. Amazingly, not only do Okinawans have long life expectancies, but they also exhibit much lower rates of heart disease and other age-related diseases (Kagawa, 1978). These are results we would expect from those practicing CR.

As you might have guessed, one major problem with CR is hunger. Unlike the Okinawans, in Western culture, restricting calories for an extended period when you're used to eating at will is difficult (if not impossible) for most people. Therefore, interest has turned toward an alternative way of reducing food intake that gives participants some relief from hunger: inter-mittent fasting.

What Is Intermittent Fasting (IF)?

As previously stated, the problem with caloric restriction is that it's tough for many people to stick with due to hunger. For this reason, intermittent fasting has been proposed as a more real-istic alternative to caloric restriction. Intermittent fasting is the practice of either dramatically reducing how much you eat or forgoing food entirely for a set period. Outside the fasting period, you eat a normal amount of calories from a variety of nutritious meals. Intermittent fasting has been lauded for its health benefits and ability to reduce the risk for many age-related health problems, including heart disease, type II diabetes, and Alzheimer's disease. Laboratory studies have found that markers for all age-related illnesses decreased when IF was introduced to an animal's diet (Mattson, Longo, and Harvie, 2017). Like caloric restriction, IF is also an effective way to lose weight.

Many different schedules are available for intermittent fasting, ranging from restricting eating to a couple of hours a day to forgoing everything but water for days. While lengthy water fasts may seem intimidating to someone not used to fasting, you won't starve to death over several days if you eat enough to nourish yourself on your eating days. The health benefits will almost certainly outweigh the discomfort you feel during your fasting days! Furthermore, IF is psychologically easier to stick to than caloric restriction, as you only feel hungry for a set period, not constantly. There is no right way to do intermittent fasting, so gather information to figure out what will work for you in consultation with your doctor.

The health benefits of IF show up in several ways. First, inter-mittent fasting creates a type of hormesis, which, you may recall, places your body under a short-term but somewhat intense level of stress. Hormesis turns on the genes in the survival circuit, which promote DNA repair by sirtuins and improved mitochondrial function due to activation of AMPK when energy is low. Furthermore, intermittent fasting allows you to benefit from *autophagy* (Mattson, Longo, and Harvie, 2017). Autophagy is a recycling process activated by the survival circuit when energy is in short supply. As a result, your cells transition to a state of self-eating, where they digest and recycle debris and toxins from the intracellular space. Current scientific data suggests that a lack of autophagy is linked to several age-related diseases, such as atherosclerosis and type II diabetes (Moulis and Vindis, 2018).

Furthermore, intermittent fasting promotes weight loss since you'll likely consume fewer calories than a person who eats on a typical schedule. In addition, sugar and carbohydrates (easily metabolized fuels) are not readily available during fasting, so your body has to work harder to convert fat into ketone bodies for fuel. When elevated levels of ketone bodies exist in the blood, this is defined as a state of ketosis.

Restricting Food Groups

Along with eating less, another great thing you can do for your anti-aging health routine is to look at the types and content of foods you eat. There are many foods worth avoiding and some you should include when you're eating to extend your lifespan. For example, your food choices can directly affect your digestive tract and, consequently, your immune system, creating problems such as leaky gut syndrome.

Leaky gut syndrome is an unpleasant condition closely linked to age and characterized by increased inflammation throughout the digestive tract. Chronic inflammation, which results from abnormal intercellular signaling, is an important marker of aging.

While leaky gut syndrome and its effects are the subjects of some controversy (Wallace, 2017), in theory, it results from a problem with the gut lining. Nutrients are usually absorbed into the bloodstream and lymph system through specialized cells in the gut lining. Leaky gut syndrome occurs when openings between cells in the gut lining create an unwanted increase in the intestinal wall's permeability. The increased permeability is an abnormal situation that allows undesirable particles to enter circulation directly, causing inflammation. "Increased intestinal permeability," as described by the medical community, is a characteristic of some gastrointestinal illnesses such as Celiac disease. However, Dr. Robert Wallace, author of *Gut Crisis*, a book that outlines the importance of a healthy gut to a person's overall well-being, believes leaky gut syndrome is a condition unto itself and is closely affected by both the gut microbiome and the foods we eat (Wallace, 2017). He believes promoting healthy gut bacteria through eating a healthy diet helps prevent leaky gut syndrome. Since inflammation contributes to aging, reducing inflammation through diet should be essential to any anti-aging lifestyle.

Below, we've included a brief list of foods you may choose to exclude from your diet and foods that would be helpful to include. Recommendations are drawn primarily from Wallace's book *Gut Crisis* and Gundry's book *The Longevity Paradox*, which explore the relationship between gut health, the gut microbiome, and aging.

Below are things you may want to avoid or eliminate, as well as healthy alternatives:

- *Sugars/Simple Carbohydrates*

As we have noted, inflammation is one of the primary drivers of aging. The incredible amount of refined sugars and simple carbohydrates (carbs) most people eat promote the inflammation underlying most age-related diseases. The simple structure of these compounds allows them to be quickly absorbed upon consumption, leading to a tsunami of sugar entering the bloodstream. Consuming high levels of sugars and simple carbohydrates, such as glucose and fructose, is linked to various age-related health problems, like type II diabetes, obesity, and heart disease (Evans, 2016). A review of the currently available nutritional and pharmacological interventions to combat aging suggests that diets with low amounts of sugar can activate genes associated with the survival circuit in imitation of fasting and cites studies demonstrating these results in animal models (Ros and Carrascosa, 2020).

Cut sugar from your diet by avoiding processed and packaged snacks, non-diet soda, candy, and desserts as much as possible. Grains are high in carbs, as well as lectins, and are also best avoided. Instead of eating grains, opt for alternative foods made from almond flour, coconut flour, and basmati rice. When it comes to sweeteners, opt for stevia, xylitol, or monk fruit. You can also bake with all of these. However, please note that xylitol is harmful to pets.

- *Artificial Sweeteners*

Given the disadvantages of eating a lot of sugar and simple carbohydrates, you might be thinking about stocking up on Splenda or another artificial sweetener to satisfy your sweet tooth. Unfortunately, these compounds can also cause adverse health effects, and it's best to restrict how much you take in or, even better, eliminate them. In his book, Gundry references *Sweet Deception: Why Splenda, Nutrasweet, and the FDA May Be Hazardous to Your Health* by Dr. Joseph Mercola, a book detailing the hidden dangers of these additives. In *Sweet Deception,* Mercola describes the widely unknown potential health effects of Splenda, the U.S.'s best-selling artificial sweetener known for its slogan, "Made from sugar, so it tastes like sugar." However, Mercola points out that sucralose, sold under the name Splenda, is made through a five-step process where sugar is chemically treated with several compounds, creating a molecule unlike anything in nature. In addition, unlike natural disaccharides (sugars made of two sugar units), Splenda does not contain any glucose, so our bodies cannot digest it. Furthermore, creating Splenda produces chlorocarbons by replacing hydrogen atoms in the sugar molecule with chlorine atoms. Since our bodies are not made to metabolize chlorine, chlorocarbons build up in our cells and damage hepatocyte cells, which filter harmful compounds in the liver (Mercola, 2006).

- *Lectins and Wheat Germ Agglutinin*

Lectins are a class of proteins that exist in a range of foods, including grains, tomatoes, beans, peanuts, and cashews. Lectins can do significant damage to your gut health. Lectins bind to carbohydrates on the surface of the cells that line the gut, interfering with normal digestion and contributing to leaky gut syndrome. This leads to increased inflammation, a clear contributor to the symptoms of aging. While you may not need to eliminate lectins from your diet, especially if you use a "lectin blocker" (see the section on supplements below), you should avoid them.

Two of the most harmful proteins commonly present in food are gluten and wheat germ agglutinin (WGA), primarily found in wheat. While gluten is not technically a lectin, it is similar due to its ability to bind to gut cells. Many people have intolerances to gluten, including those who have Celiac disease, characterized by an immune response caused by increased intestinal permeability. Even if you don't have a severe gluten intolerance, WGA can cause digestive problems in many people. One study in 2009 showed that WGA could increase intestinal permeability to dextran and mannitol, common compounds found in foods, leading to an inflammatory reaction when these compounds pass through the gut barrier (Pellegrina et al., 2009).

- *Foods With Pesticides*

Pesticides are chemical compounds sprayed onto crops to repel or kill off pests like insects and rodents. Natural eating guides strongly recommend choosing organic foods or those grown without chemical pesticides, but does this really affect your gut health? According to Wallace in *Gut Crisis* (2017), avoiding foods treated with pesticides is not just a fad but an essential factor in creating a healthy diet. While Wallace links his recommendation to avoid pesticides to *Ayurveda*, a philosophical viewpoint on healthy living and medicine from the Indian subcontinent, scientific data supports the notion that pesticides in food can harm a person's health. For example, two reviews of the evidence around pesticide consumption and neurodegenerative diseases revealed that a high amount of pesticides in the diet could increase a person's risk of Alzheimer's and Parkinson's diseases, both progressive age-related illnesses (Ahmed et al., 2017) (Yan et al., 2016). In addition, a common herbicide used in farming called RoundUp has some adverse effects on gut bacteria. This herbicide contains a chemical known as glyphosate, which disrupts the balance of gut bacteria and inhibits their ability to synthesize hormones and other biochemicals our bodies need. This disruption can also contribute to inflammation and leaky gut syndrome, allowing pathogens to gain a foothold in the gut (Samsel and Seneff, 2013). Since grains and beans high in lectins are commonly treated with RoundUp, your body gets an inflammatory "double whammy" from consuming these foods!

On the other hand, organic farms use more natural biopesticides to protect plants from pests. Regardless, you should always thoroughly wash produce before eating it to remove any compounds added at the farm. Anyone looking to avoid age-related health problems should choose organic foods whenever possible.

- *Meat and Animal Products*

While meat and other animal products, such as dairy and eggs, are packed with proteins and other nutrients, they may do more harm than good.

Currently, most of our meat is produced on factory farms. Animals, such as pigs, chickens, and milk cows, are kept in cramped and crowded conditions for most of their extremely stressful lives. Using antibiotics to stave off disease in animals or hormones to promote growth are the usual practices of these farms. However, in *The Longevity Paradox,* Gundry points out that these compounds could disrupt human gut bacteria, reducing their diversity and harming gut health. So unless you can find and consume antibiotic-free and hormone-free meat or milk, the food you're eating may have small amounts of antibiotics and hormones, which pass into your system during digestion!

While protein is good for you and essential for life, it's also possible to have too much protein. Wallace cites Mercola in his description of this problem. People with a heavy meat diet are likely taking in too much of the amino acid *methionine.* Large amounts of methionine can activate mTOR, part of your cells' nutrient-sensing apparatuses that promotes growth when there's plenty of protein available. As inhibition of mTOR is linked to autophagy and other anti-aging processes, it's worth avoiding its activation when possible. Plant-based foods have lower levels of methionine than animal foods (Sinclair, 2019). Therefore, including plant-based proteins in your diet is the healthier choice.

Given the potential health problems of animal-based foods, Sinclair points out that there is not a single amino acid found in meat and other animal products that is not also found in plants. In addition, a lower protein diet can help trigger the survival circuit through hormesis, supporting good health. So again, choosing plant-based foods can help reduce your risk of age-related diseases associated with eating meat and animal products.

Finally, another potentially harmful compound from animal products is casein A1, found in most dairy. Both casein A1 and A2 are proteins in milk and products made from milk. However, casein A1 can cause digestive discomfort and higher rates of inflammation, a significant contributor to age-related health problems (Jianquin et al., 2016). According to Gundry, casein A1 converts to an opioid peptide during digestion and then binds to insulin-producing cells, causing an inflammatory immune reaction (Gundry, 2019). While you don't need to give up dairy entirely, reducing your dairy intake or choosing casein A2 dairy products (available at some health stores) can help avoid the inflammation caused by casein A1. Most dairy products from cows in the US contain casein A1, unlike those from cows bred in some European countries that are more likely to have casein A2.

- *Oils*

Some oils are good for your health. For example, olive oil is packed with polyphenols and healthy unsaturated fats and can be essential to a healthy anti-aging diet. However, other oils can have significant adverse health effects and are thus better avoided.

Hydrogenated oils have had hydrogen added through an artificial process. This supposed advancement in food science allows the storage of high-calorie foods without refrigeration. Unfortunately, hydrogenation also created trans fats, which have been recognized as generally harmful for some time. As a result, the FDA mandated in 2015 that fully hydrogenated oils be phased out of foods by 2018 (FDA, 2015). However, partially hydrogenated oils are still used in commercially fried foods, treats made with shortening such as cookies or donuts, and packaged snacks.

The ill effects of trans fats are also well-known. They can raise blood levels of undesirable LDL cholesterol, leading to an increased risk of age-related illnesses, including heart disease and type II diabetes (American Heart Association, 2021). Trans fats are another reason why one should avoid processed, prepackaged foods. Also, beware that trans fats are present in animal products, especially red meat.

- *Fruits in Excess*

The vitamins and fiber in fruit are essential aspects of a healthy diet. Therefore, in *Gut Crisis* Wallace recommends eating fruit as part of your gut-healthy diet, especially when you're recovering from eating something harmful to your gut bacteria. However, consuming fruits in moderation is important because of their naturally high sugar content.

According to Gundry in *The Longevity Paradox,* much of the sugar in fruits comes from fructose, which is more difficult than glucose for your small intestine to absorb. Fructose is also associated with mitochondrial dysfunction. One study in rats demonstrated that a high-fructose diet could harm mitochondrial DNA and reduce mitochondrial biogenesis (Cioffi et al., 2017). A review of human studies showed that excessive intake of fructose increases the risk of type II diabetes, hypertension, and other metabolic health problems (Kretowicz et al., 2011).

Fruits are essential to a healthy diet, but being mindful of how much fruit you're eating and not overdoing your intake can help you avoid the adverse effects of high levels of fructose in your system.

Things to incorporate into a healthy diet:

Apart from the unhealthy foods we've just discussed and some healthy alternatives, below we offer more healthy choices that one can add to their diet, including a number of anti-aging supplements.

- *Plenty of Water*

Hydration is vital to any healthy lifestyle, and routines intended to reduce the effects of aging on the body are no exception. Water is essential to every single process in the human body, and it makes up between 55-75% of our body mass (depending on our age). So, not getting enough water can be highly disruptive to the function of cells, organs, and tissues. In addition, according to an extensive review of the effects of good and poor hydration on all age groups, good hydration is linked to a lower risk of some forms of heart disease (hypertension and fatal coronary heart disease) and hyperglycemia in diabetic ketoacidosis, a dangerous condition suffered by individuals with type II diabetes (Popkin, D'Anci and Rosenberg, 2010). Also, being dehydrated can make you feel hungry and lethargic, making it harder to stick to other anti-aging lifestyle practices like eating a healthy diet and exercising.

Best practices suggest taking approximately 64 ounces of water daily, the equivalent of 8 cups. Along with drinking glasses of water, tea, or coffee, you can also increase your water intake by eating foods high in this essential substance, such as celery and lettuce.

- *Foods That Promote Gut Health*

Throughout *The Longevity Paradox,* Dr. Steven Gundry provides several lists of foods that promote gut health, reduce inflammation, and improve digestion for overall well-being. Eating these foods can help nourish your gut microbiome, allowing them to produce the metabolites that keep the cells of your digestive tract strong and healthy. While a full exploration of the benefits of these foods would take up much more space than we have available in this book, we've included some of Gundry's food recommendations with notes on their potential benefits.

Prebiotic foods are foods high in fiber. They are broken down by gut microbiota into short-chain fatty acids, the primary energy source for essential cells lining the gut wall. High-fiber, prebiotic foods recommended by Gundry include ground flaxseed, cruciferous vegetables, artichokes, leeks, okra, chicory, nuts, and mushrooms.

Gundry also recommends eating low-sugar fruits, especially those without seeds, because fruits with seeds typically contain lectins. Low-sugar fruits are not only high in fiber but also packed with vitamins. Among these many fruits, avocados are unique because they also have healthy unsaturated fats. Other low-sugar fruits on Gundry's list include green bananas, green pears, berries, figs, and coconuts.

Foods high in healthy fats are highly recommended by Gundry, as they reduce inflammation and may also have cognitive benefits. These include perilla seed oil, olive oil, MCT oil, coconut oil, walnut oil, and avocado oil.

Anti-Aging Supplements

Taking supplements might sound straightforward, but they can be trickier than you think. One of the problems is that supplements are not regulated, and in many cases not well-studied.

So, we thought it would be good to provide you with our personal experience with supplements— the good, the bad, and the ugly.

John's Experience With Anti-Aging Supplements:

I've been taking supplements as part of my health routine for decades and have had some interesting experiences. I'll share one example in particular. I noticed something strange when I added CBD oil and Lion's Mane mushrooms to my diet. My hair was no longer getting caught in the drain when I showered. I simply wasn't losing it. Lisa noticed too and asked if I was growing more hair on my head. At first, I told her I didn't know, but before long, it was impossible to deny. I'm not sure which of the supplements were reducing my hair loss and promoting hair growth or if it was a combination of both, but they were the only two new additions to my diet at the time. Go figure…

Lisa's Experience With Anti-Aging Supplements:

I am one of those people who jumps into things with both feet, and I took on supplementation the same way. While I have really benefited from supplementation overall, I have also run into a few glitches. The first glitch I ran into was trying a lithium supplement sold by a company that cites loads of research on its website. I read the research on the anti-aging benefits of taking low-dose lithium and decided to start taking it without my nurse practitioner's knowledge (am I bad?). Subsequently, after a few months, I felt something funny in my heart. I was so scared I went to see my nurse practitioner and then a specialist. The specialist recommended I wear a heart monitor for a day or so. The monitoring showed that I had a heart rhythm with rare "premature ventricular contractions" (PVCs) and rare "premature atrial contractions" (PACs), whatever that means. My nurse practitioner said that these conditions, in my case, were "nothing to worry about." However, I was not pleased with this diagnosis because I had never had this before, so I began my research.

Sure enough, I eventually focused on the lithium I was taking and discovered it could sometimes affect your heart rhythm. Why wasn't that on the label? So, that was it for me and lithium. I stopped taking it, and after a few weeks, I had no more funny feelings in my heart— the arrhythmia had disappeared. Thank God!

The second glitch I encountered was getting too large a dose of certain supplements without realizing it. I found that some of the supplements I was taking, like melatonin, also had a B vitamin that I was already getting from my B vitamin supplement. I found the same thing with two other supplements I was taking; both had added B vitamins. Consequently, I was overdosing on B vitamins. I believe the excessive doses of niacin (B3) gave me what I called "the itchies," in which I felt itchy on my face, back of my neck, and arms. When I lowered my B vitamin intake, "the itchies" disappeared and my bloodwork that had shown high B12 had returned to normal.

What did I learn? Well, for one, I need to read all the ingredients in my supplements to ensure I'm not getting too much of a good thing. Secondly, I need and want my doctor or nurse practitioner's input if I try something a little off the beaten track, like lithium. Thirdly, I learned how valuable it is to have bloodwork done regularly because it gives you a quantitative health assessment. For example, I realized that getting too much Biotin (B6) can skew the values of some bloodwork test results. I found this bit of knowledge in medical literature after being prompted by an annotation in my bloodwork results asking about my biotin intake. So, I cut down my biotin intake and suggest that anyone taking biotin be aware of its impact on some types of bloodwork. If in doubt, talk to your doctor or nurse practitioner. Finally, from these experiences, I learned how important it was to do my own research and share it with my nurse practitioner, along with any questions.

The supplements listed here have shown some promise based on research to combat at least some of the hallmarks of aging. Note that supplements are not a quick fix to the problem of aging: You can't expect a supplement regimen on its own to make a real improvement without making lifestyle changes as well. However, in many cases, supplements can be a scientifically sound way to complement your healthy lifestyle choices and give your anti-aging health routine the extra push it needs to reach its full potential.

Not every supplement is suitable for everyone. As always, you should talk to your doctor or nurse practitioner before starting a supplement regimen. Before you start, a medical professional could point out potential medication conflicts or other concerns.

- **Probiotics**

Probiotics are foods that contain live colonies of the bacteria that live in our guts. The idea of eating live bacteria might be distasteful to some, but, likely, you've already been eating probiotic foods. For example, fermented foods like kombucha, sauerkraut, and kimchi contain live bacterial colonies. Furthermore, yogurt or other dairy products, such as kefir, contain probiotics. Probiotics are also available as a powder you can mix into drinks or food. If you add probiotics to your diet, follow the package directions for how much to consume to ensure you get the full benefits.

In *The Longevity Paradox*, Gundry points out that most of the probiotics we take through food are destroyed by stomach acid (though some make it to the gut). To rectify this problem and ensure you get the most out of your probiotic intake, Gundry markets Bio Complete 3. Like other effective probiotics, it contains *Bacillus coagulans*, or BC30, a spore-forming species of bacteria not digested by stomach acid that can make its way to the lower intestine intact (Gundry, 2019). Finally, in *Gut Crisis*, Robert Wallace agrees that oral probiotics can be helpful but reminds the reader that they will likely have to continue taking a high dose of probiotics over an extended period to receive the full benefits.

Remember, once these helpful critters are in your gut, they need to be fed to grow, multiply, and become a permanent part of your gut microbiome. Eating a high-fiber diet with plenty of prebiotic foods will ensure that the probiotics you consume will be there to stay.

- **Prebiotics**

Prebiotics are often confused with probiotics. Many people don't even realize that these are two separate things (for example, the computer this book was written on attempted to auto-correct *prebiotics* to *probiotics*). However, prebiotics and probiotics benefit your gut health in separate ways, and being aware of the difference can help you optimize your dietary choices to support your gut health.

As we established in *The Importance of the Gut Microbiome*, helpful gut bacteria digest the long-chain fibrous carbohydrates in your diet that you can't, producing several metabolites that support your gut health. For example, several species of gut bacteria produce *butyrate*, a short-chain fatty acid used for energy by the cells in your large intestine. Butyrate also combats obesity and may even improve your brain health (see the dedicated section on butyrate below for more information on how this works). According to Gundry, eating plenty of prebiotic foods helps support your gut bacteria by ensuring they have the nutrition they need to grow and divide, keeping their population at a healthy level.

So what foods are prebiotic? While you can purchase yogurts or other foods with prebiotics added, you can also get them naturally from select foods. Among a long list of healthy foods with prebiotic properties is ground flaxseed, which is high in fiber and polyphenols, B vitamins, and long-chain Omega 3s. Other foods that Gundry suggests eating for their prebiotic properties are cruciferous vegetables, artichokes, chicory, mushrooms, yams and tubers, leeks, okra, endives, and nuts. And you can always get prebiotics in supplement form.

- **Butyrate**

As we just mentioned, butyrate is a short-chain fatty acid produced by some species of gut bacteria—but only certain species, which is one reason why the diversity of your gut microbiome is key to good digestive health. Gundry also notes butyrate is an excellent way to combat the negative effects of what he calls a "365-day growth cycle." This year-long growth cycle exists when rich foods are constantly available and the body rarely, if ever, undergoes a period of fasting or eating less. Butyrate dampens this growth cycle and protects against obesity and type II diabetes in part by promoting inefficient metabolism (Mollica et al., 2017). Essentially, butyrate causes mitochondria to work less efficiently, so the rate of metabolism needs to increase to generate the same level of energy. Therefore, cells function as if less nutrition is available (i.e., fasting). In other words, butyrate mimics the effects of fasting. The Mollica study demonstrated how butyrate or a synthetic equivalent could protect against the consequences of obesity and type II diabetes, specifically fatty liver and insulin resistance. Fatty liver, also known as hepatic steatosis, is a condition where excess fat builds up in the liver, causing inflammation, scarring, and potentially liver failure. Mice fed a diet containing extra natural or synthetic butyrate showed a massive improvement in their symptoms. Specifically, the researchers noted a decline in the level of lipids, or fats, accumulating in these mice's livers over the course of the experiment. Not only that, but the mice supplemented with butyrate were better able to regulate their blood sugar than the control group, suggesting their insulin resistance was also in decline (Mollica et al., 2017).

The mitochondria-boosting properties of butyrate may also improve brain function. A review of the evidence suggests that a high-fiber diet can improve brain function because it supports a healthy gut microbiome. Bourassa et al. postulate that butyrate may interact directly with the central nervous system. They point out that while most butyrate produced in the gut is consumed for energy by colonocytes (the cells that make up the inner layer of the gut wall) or absorbed into the liver, a portion escapes and circulates in the bloodstream (Bourassa et al., 2016). They also reference a 2014 study that used mice engineered to be born without gut microbiota. The blood-brain barrier of these mice had an unhealthy permeability, potentially letting unwanted compounds into the brain. However, upon introducing butyrate-producing bacteria into these mice, the permeability of the blood-brain barrier returned to a normal level. Besides that, colonizing the mice with butyrate-producing bacteria increased the acetylation of histones in brain cells. Recalling that histones are responsible for packaging DNA, the study results suggest that butyrate has a protective, epigenetic effect on the brain (Braniste et al., 2014). There is already evidence that this effect translates to humans—children on high-fiber diets show better cognition than their counterparts on poorer diets (Khan et al., 2015).

• **Polyphenols**

Polyphenols are a broad range of naturally occurring compounds that can boost digestion by supporting your gut microbiome's health. They may also stimulate genes associated with longevity and the survival circuit. Furthermore, gut bacteria convert polyphenols into anti-inflammatory compounds as they digest them, helping to combat inflammation in the brain and throughout the body (Gundry, 2019).

One of the most well-known polyphenols is epigallocatechin gallate (EGCG). You've probably seen articles lauding the health benefits of green tea, and this compound is responsible for many of them. EGCG has been shown to trigger the production of more mitochondria in cells, restoring mitochondrial function that may have been in decline. In addition, EGCG stimulates AMPK and SIRT1, which promote longevity (Xiong et al., 2018). To add this compound to your daily routine, you can take a tablet supplement of EGCG or regularly drink green tea.

Olive oil and olives are also excellent sources of polyphenols and a great source of healthy fats. The polyphenols in olive oil, the most prominent of which is oleuropein, help to protect against heart disease, Alzheimer's disease, and other age-related diseases by stimulating autophagy and other beneficial processes. The anti-inflammatory effect of oleuropein comes from its inhibition of leukotriene B4, an inflammatory mediator produced by macrophages. It also inhibits the activity of lipoxygenase enzymes that create inflammatory mediators. Finally, oleuropein has anti-cancer effects by inhibiting the growth and viability of several types of tumor cells (Omar,

2010). You can increase the amount of oleuropein in your diet by using olive oil as a cooking oil and in sauces and dressings as much as possible or by taking a supplement in tablet form.

- **Resveratrol**

Resveratrol is likely the most important of the polyphenols commonly found in food. You've probably heard people say that red wine is good for your heart, and resveratrol is cited as the cause of this cardioprotective effect (Baur and Sinclair, 2006). In addition, another study has shown that resveratrol induces autophagy by activating sirtuins (Morselli et al., 2011), suggesting that it has a longevity-promoting effect similar to caloric restriction (Sinclair, 2019).

So how does resveratrol work its magic? According to an extensive study by Morselli et al. in 2011, resveratrol activates autophagy primarily through directly or indirectly activating SIRT1, a sirtuin that acts as a *deacetylase* (among its other roles). Deacetylases remove acetyl groups from other compounds, which can change the way they function and interact with other compounds. Activating SIRT1 in the cytoplasm (the space inside a cell where organelles reside) sets off a cascade of biochemical interactions that induce autophagy (Morselli et al., 2011). While the study was inconclusive as to whether resveratrol activates SIRT1 directly or indirectly, Morselli et al. did establish that resveratrol is a potent inducer of autophagy through the SIRT1 pathway.

The Morselli et al. study also demonstrated that a combination of resveratrol and a polyamine called spermidine could activate autophagy at a lower dose than either could activate the process alone (Morselli et al., 2011). Polyamines are found in a wide range of foods, from leafy greens and cruciferous vegetables to nuts and seeds, to fermented foods like kimchi, as well as lentils, chicken liver, aged cheeses, and mushrooms.

- **AMPK Metabolic Activator**

As previously mentioned, adenosine monophosphate protein kinase (AMPK) is a cellular compound involved in the same cascade of chemical reactions as SIRT1 and other biochemical products of longevity genes. Like sirtuins and RNA polymerase, AMPK is an enzyme that facilitates biochemical reactions that would otherwise not be possible. The primary role of AMPK is to restore function to the mitochondria when energy is limited, such as during fasting or caloric restriction. Activating this pathway helps raise cellular NAD+ levels, combat mitochondrial dysfunction, and switch on a number of additional genes that promote survival and longevity (Sinclair, 2019).

Adenosine monophosphate (AMP) is a small cellular compound that interacts with AMPK in the cytoplasm. When these compounds bind, AMPK undergoes a *conformational change*, or a change in shape that switches it to its active form. There are two sites on AMPK where AMP can bind. The first site can be bound only by AMP, while AMP, adenosine diphosphate (ADP), and adenosine triphosphate (ATP), the energy molecule produced by metabolism, compete to bind to the second site. AMPK is turned off when ATP binds to the second site, indicating that energy is available to the cell. When AMP binds to the first site, this indicates that energy is less abundant, turning on AMPK and triggering the survival circuit. Remember, the survival circuit signals the cell to repair DNA damage that would otherwise shorten the organism's lifespan. If AMP or ADP binds to the second site, this induces a conformational change that prevents ATP from blocking AMPK activation (Xiao et al., 2013). Supplementing with a chemical mimic of AMP can help activate inactive AMPK residing in the cytoplasm, triggering the rest of the AMPK-SIRT1 pathway (Kim et al., 2016). In short, studies suggest that taking an AMPK metabolic activator as a supplement may support DNA repair and promote longevity.

- **NAD+**

NADH, and its oxidized form NAD+, is a molecule essential to your body's production of energy in the form of ATP from glucose and other nutrients. It also plays a vital role in DNA repair and gene expression. NAD+ is required for the proper functioning of sirtuins and is part of the survival circuit that promotes longevity in our cells, similar to fasting or other forms of hormesis. Cellular levels of NAD+ decrease with age, leading to mitochondrial dysfunction and an increased risk of genomic instability (Sinclair, 2019). Furthermore, boosting NAD+ stimulates SIRT1 to action, suppressing mTOR and creating an effect similar to fasting, where genes associated with the survival circuit are active and working to protect the cell. Therefore, it's not surprising that someone looking for an anti-aging supplement would look into ways to boost their cellular level of NAD+. The most accessible NAD+ booster on the market is nicotinamide riboside (NR).

A recent (2020) review by Mehmel, Jovanovic, and Spitz gives an extensive overview of the evidence for the anti-aging effects of NR supplementation. As both NAD+ depletion and mitochondrial dysfunction are linked to the onset of Alzheimer's and other age-related neurodegenerative diseases, NR can help prevent the development of these illnesses by raising NAD+ levels in the cell (Kerr et al., 2017). In addition, increased levels of NAD+ boost mitochondrial function and promote DNA repair by sirtuins (Mehmel, Jovanovic, and Spitz, 2020), combating genomic instability. NR supplementation has also been shown to increase NAD+ levels and, thus, sirtuin activation like caloric restriction (Belenky et al., 2007), suggesting that NR supplementation can provide health benefits even when you're not restricting calories.

• **Vitamins and Minerals**

Vitamins and minerals are diverse groups of small molecules that play essential roles in cellular function. While they only need to be consumed in small amounts, vitamin and mineral deficiencies are unfortunately very common, especially among people who are malnourished or eat a diet primarily of packaged foods. While eating a varied diet rich in fruits and vegetables satisfies most people's vitamin and mineral requirements, others can benefit from vitamin and mineral supplements. Studies have shown that a number of vitamins and minerals are crucial to health and worth considering as part of your anti-aging supplement routine.

While you've probably heard of vitamin B, there is a range of B vitamins with different but related effects. Gut bacteria primarily produce these, but many can also be found in foods. According to Gundry, many people have deficiencies, especially in *methylcobalamin*, the active form of vitamin B12, and *methyl folate*, the active form of folic acid. Many people also carry an MTHFR gene mutation that harms their ability to make these vitamins. In *The Longevity Paradox*, Gundry suggests taking a B vitamin supplement, as many people have elevated levels of the amino acid homocysteine in their bloodstream, which can damage the inner linings of blood vessels. Taking a B vitamin supplement helps return blood concentrations of homocysteine to healthy levels by converting excess amounts of this amino acid to a neutral compound that does not harm the blood vessels. Gundry recommends taking a daily dose of 1,000 mcg of methyl folate and 1,000 to 5,000 mcg of methyl B12 sublingually (under the tongue).

Vitamin C is vital for the body's ability to repair collagen, the most common protein in our bodies. Collagen is a major structural component of skin, blood vessels, and connective tissue; therefore, to keep your body in top shape, it's essential to have plenty of vitamin C in your system. Being out in the sun allows UV radiation to damage the collagen in your skin, but vitamin C promotes repair, keeping skin looking and feeling younger. As vitamin C is water-soluble and quickly excreted in the urine, Gundry recommends a time-released supplement to reap the benefits of the vitamin before it's expelled.

Vitamin D3 helps activate stem cells in your gut, which are essential for combating damage or degradation of the intestinal lining due to poor diet or inflammation. Keeping the intestinal lining in good shape promotes nutrient absorption, letting you get the most out of everything you eat and reducing gastrointestinal issues. Furthermore, vitamin D3 is linked to improved proteostasis, while deficient levels are associated with age-related diseases, including Alzheimer's, Parkinson's, and cancer, where accumulating misfolded proteins may play a role (Mark et al., 2016). Therefore, Gundry highly recommends that his patients take 5,000 IU of vitamin D3 in supplements daily. While this number may seem high, toxicity from vitamin D3 is very rare, as the body has a high storage capacity for the vitamin (Marcinowska-Suchowierska et al., 2018).

Vitamin K2 is essential because it helps your blood clot correctly when you're injured. Along with its role in blood clotting, vitamin K2 is necessary for regulating calcium deposition in your body. It increases the calcification of the bones while preventing calcium from building up in the blood vessels and kidneys. Calcification of the arteries is troublesome because it is linked to heart disease, one of the most prominent age-related diseases. For example, one study of approximately 4,800 people over 10-years-old showed that a higher vitamin K2 intake was associated with a lower risk of dying of heart disease (Geleijnse et al., 2004). There may also be benefits to your bone health. A review of the link between vitamin K intake and bone fractures indicated that taking vitamin K2 may reduce the loss of bone density as people age, thus reducing their chances of fractures (Cockayne et al., 2006).

Another concern is that the mineral content of food has declined. The first reason is that foods are now grown in soils that have become mineral-depleted. In turn, meat and dairy products can also be depleted of nutrients, especially minerals, because animals eat grasses and grains grown in mineral-depleted soil. Secondly, when foods are processed and packaged with addictive additives and harmful dyes, the nutrient content is diluted and thus further diminished (Thomas, 2007). A review of the literature by the National Institute on Aging suggests that older adults can benefit from more calcium (which combats loss of bone density associated with age) and magnesium (which promotes protein synthesis and muscle repair). If you're an older adult concerned about frailty, consider foods fortified with minerals. Research findings suggest increasing potassium intake because it provides a broad range of benefits, including enhancing metabolism, supporting protein synthesis, improving muscle function, and regulating the heartbeat (National Institute on Aging, 2021).

- **Baby Aspirin**

Aspirin is an over-the-counter medication to treat pain, fevers, and swelling. Aspirin also interferes with the process of blood clotting. While this seems undesirable, taking a low-dose baby aspirin can help prevent heart attacks and strokes by preventing blood clots from blocking important arteries or reaching the brain, especially in adults with cardiac issues. The correct dose to take each day has been widely debated and may depend on the individual's gender, age, and history of cardiac problems. One review of the evidence for aspirin's ability to prevent cardiac events and which doses were effective for different populations suggests that 160 mg per day is ideal for most people. However, 75 mg per day has been effective in patients with stable coronary artery disease (Dalen, 2006).

Furthermore, taking 81 mg of enteric-coated aspirin daily can help trigger EPA and DPA, the omega-3 fatty acids found in fish, to reduce inflammation in your nerves and eyes. It does this by activating the creation of *resolvins*, potent anti-inflammatory molecules, from the omega-3s (Dalli et al., 2013). However, remember that it's always a good idea to talk to your doctor before starting any new medication.

- **Lectin Blockers**

Recall that lectins are proteins found in wheat, tomatoes, beans, and other grains, fruits, and vegetables that bind to carbohydrates on the surface of the intestinal lining, interfering with digestion, promoting leaky gut syndrome, and increasing inflammation. Luckily, some compounds can bind to lectins to negate their effects before they wreak havoc on our digestive systems. Two examples of lectin-binding supplements are glucosamine and methylsulfonylmethane (MSM). These are useful if you accidentally eat something with more lectins than you intended or have no choice but to eat a high-lectin meal when someone else cooks for you!

Glucosamine, scientifically known by its full chemical name *N-acetyl-D-glucosamine*, has been shown to bind to lectins in a laboratory environment. One study even proposes using it as a model when studying the binding specificity of different lectins

(Cederberg and Gray, 1979). As well as using glucosamine and MSM as lectin blockers, people also choose to use them for other anti-aging reasons because they can combat osteoarthritis, a common inflammatory age-related illness characterized by painful joints. Glucosamine is used by the body to synthesize critical structural components in the joints, allowing the body to repair osteoarthritis damage (Reginster et al., 2012). While MSM is used by the body to repair connective tissues, it also has anti-inflammatory properties (Kim et al., 2006). As you may recall, John found relief for his arthritic hip from Bi-Flex, which contains both glucosamine and MSM. He didn't know it then, but he was also promoting good gut health.

- **Senolytics**

The term "lysis" is commonly used in cell biology to refer to destroying a cell by breaking its cell membrane. A class of compounds known as senolytics seeks out and destroys senescent cells. The destruction of senescent cells helps combat two hallmarks of aging: the accumulation of senescent cells and their abnormal intracellular signaling. Senolytics kill senescent cells by triggering their removal and preventing them from secreting undesirable inflammatory "panic" signals. As senescent cells do not undergo apoptosis (cell disintegration) like healthy cells do at the end of their lifespan, several drugs have been developed to target senescent cells specifically without harming the healthy cells nearby.

Senolytics make up a new class of drugs, and research into their efficacy in combating age-related diseases is ongoing. However, there is already evidence testifying to their potential benefits. Some examples of these compounds include fisetin, quercetin, nobiletin, and spermidine. One of the most easily accessible senolytics is fisetin, derived from a compound found in fruits, vegetables, nuts, and wine. According to the current scientific research, a review of the benefits of fisetin shows that it has strong anti-inflammatory properties in humans and animals (Pal, Pearlman, and Afaq, 2016), making it helpful in combating a number of age-related diseases like type II diabetes and heart disease. The reason that fisetin is so good at reducing inflammation is likely related to its remarkable ability to clear senescent cells. A mouse trial showed that fisetin was a more potent senolytic than nine other compounds investigated by the study. These researchers also suggested fisetin could combat age-related diseases (Yousefzadeh, 2018).

• **Berberine**

Berberine is a compound found in many plants, including the Oregon grape. The main reason you might want to have berberine in your supplement routine is its purported ability to help control blood sugar and lipid metabolism, thereby combating insulin resistance and other symptoms of type II diabetes. But is there any evidence for this?

As a matter of fact, some studies suggest that berberine is very good at controlling blood sugar in people with insulin resistance. In a double-blind study, people with type II diabetes were treated with either berberine or the established medication Metformin. Berberine was approximately as effective as

Metformin at reducing blood sugar and triglycerides, risk factors for heart disease. In another trial of the same study, people with poorly controlled type II diabetes were given berberine as a supplement. Results showed that the supplement effectively lowered blood glucose, triglycerides, and total cholesterol, especially harmful LDL cholesterol (Yin, Xing, and Ye, 2009). While the action mechanism is still under investigation, these studies suggest that berberine can be helpful to people who struggle with dysregulated nutrient sensing in the form of insulin resistance and people with high cholesterol.

- **Curcumin**

You're probably familiar with turmeric, a staple of most people's spice racks, but you may not know its potential anti-aging properties! These advantageous properties, and the spice's characteristic bright yellow color, come from the naturally produced polyphenol curcumin.

Curcumin activates several genes connected to longevity, including AMPK and sirtuins. Furthermore, it has anti-inflammatory properties that combat the effects of the molecules secreted by dysfunctional senescent cells, thereby preventing nearby healthy cells from turning into "zombies" (more senescent cells). Curcumin also holds the unique status as one of the rare compounds that can pass through the brain-blood barrier, combating inflammation in the brain and helping people who suffer from age-related cognitive decline. In *The Longevity Paradox*, Gundry describes a study where a group of people who supplemented their diets with curcumin displayed improvements in their memory recall and attention span after 18 months, compared to a control group who took a placebo (Small et al., 2018).

You can purchase curcumin as a supplement, but you can also benefit from using turmeric in your food regularly. However, there is one issue with consuming curcumin; very little actually gets absorbed when turmeric is eaten alone. Luckily, black pepper is an effective way to enhance the bioavailability of curcumin and ensure you get the full benefits. So when you use turmeric in your food, add plenty of black pepper and check that any turmeric supplement you buy also contains black pepper!

- **Green Plant Phytochemicals**

Leafy greens such as spinach, lettuce, kale, arugula, watercress, Swiss chard, and yu choy are all excellent for your gut microbiome because of their high amount of fiber. However, Gundry recommends supplementing with green plant phytochemicals to ensure your helpful gut bacteria get all the nutrition they need. Phytochemicals are bioactive compounds produced by plants, and many have health benefits for people and animals that consume them. Unfortunately, as the typical Western diet is low in greens, you likely need more phytochemicals.

Most green plant phytochemical supplements contain wheat grass and oat grass. However, these are high in harmful lectins, so be on the lookout for a supplement without them. One option could be a supplement of spinach extract, which is high in thylakoids, a phytochemical involved in photosynthesis.

Spinach extract supplements have been shown to reduce inflammation and lower blood sugar. Along with these health benefits, spinach extract can also help you lose weight by reducing your appetite (Roberts and Moreau, 2016). Weight loss can occur because thylakoids lower the levels of the hunger hormone ghrelin and interfere with fat digestion. Consequently, since fat digests more slowly, it extends the length of time the body secretes other hormones that make you feel full in response to the presence of fat (Albertsson et al., 2007).

- **Glucose Control Supplements**

A range of supplements on the market purports to help you control your blood sugar or protect your body against the effects of too much sugar. These are sold under monikers like "glucose control" or "sugar limiting." But how do they work?

Glucose control supplements limit the function of the "insulin-related growth factor" (IGF-1), an important intracellular signaling protein that impacts the rate at which your cells grow and divide. IGF-1 also plays a part in stress responses, such as hunger, and is linked to the mTOR nutrient-sensing pathway. When mTOR senses plenty of available protein and sugar, it stimulates the production of IGF-1, which encourages cell growth. When the supply of these nutrients is low, IGF-1 is inhibited. While you want IGF-1 to be active *sometimes*, promoting cell growth without a break can be dangerous. If a cell has become defective due to genomic instability or other hallmarks of aging, it may begin to grow and divide at an increased rate, which can lead to the formation of tumors. Unlimited levels of IGF-1 are dangerous because a downward spiral of epigenomic instability occurs when the body never enters autophagy, a process where defective cells are cleared away. In a gardening analogy, it's like focusing a lot of energy on growing a garden without addressing the overgrowth of weeds.

Glucose control supplements inhibit IGF-1 by working to help manage your body's absorption and processing of sugar. Remember that these supplements don't claim to manage diabetes but do help your body maintain insulin sensitivity before you start having problems. These supplements contain a wide range of compounds, but some common ingredients are chromium, zinc, selenium, and cinnamon bark extract, all of which can help you regulate blood sugar.

Chromium is a mineral that our bodies use to help control blood sugar. Our bodies have an ideal, natural level of chromium, but levels decline as we age, progressively increasing our risk of insulin resistance and related problems. However, recent studies have shown that regular supplementation with chromium can boost the metabolic action of insulin in your body and counter the effects of insulin resistance. For example, one trial had volunteers eat yeast supplemented with chromium while going about their daily lives and regular eating patterns, while another group consumed a placebo. The blood sugar of the group supplemented with chromium was significantly lower than that of the group receiving the placebo (Sharma et al., 2011).

Zinc, another essential mineral commonly included in glucose control supplements, has more robust evidence for its efficacy. Zinc supports insulin action by binding to insulin receptors, triggering cells to take up glucose from the blood. People who are deficient in zinc are at an increased risk for insulin resistance and type II diabetes than people who have enough zinc in their diets (Vashum et al., 2013). Taking a supplement is an easy way to ensure you're getting enough.

Selenium is a lesser-known mineral and element found in the Earth's soil, which is how it makes its way into water and food. While most people aren't aware that they're deficient in selenium, not getting enough of this important mineral can increase your risk of getting diseases ranging from HIV to Crohn's disease. The health benefits of selenium are still being studied, but it's already been shown to be effective in controlling blood sugar. In 2010, a study on older people at risk for blood sugar problems in France showed that selenium could help regulate blood sugar to a significant extent in men, though the effect was much weaker in women. The study didn't identify the action mechanism, but the researchers did determine the effect wasn't due to selenium acting as an antioxidant (Akbaraly et al., 2010).

Cinnamon bark extract is exactly what it sounds like—a substance extracted from the bark of the cinnamon plant—and it can dramatically reduce the effects of insulin resistance. When you see rolled-up, whole cinnamon "sticks," you're looking at cinnamon bark. A 2011 review of the effects of cinnamon bark extract suggested that the supplement can reduce fasting blood glucose in people with diabetes or prediabetes (Davis and Yokoyama, 2011). These results were corroborated by a study by Anderson et al. in 2016, where supplementation with cinnamon bark extract reduced fasting blood glucose in a group of non-diabetic volunteers.

A range of compounds is available as supplements to protect against insulin resistance or help manage existing insulin resistance. If you want to avoid taking four more daily supplements, many formulations on the market combine these compounds into one supplement. For example, Steven Gundry developed a glucose control supplement called Sugar Defense, which includes chromium, selenium, zinc, and cinnamon bark extract. Sugar Defense also contains berberine, curcumin, and black pepper, discussed in more detail in the sections above.

- **Long-Chain Omega 3s**

Omega-3 fatty acids are unsaturated fats in foods such as salmon and other fatty fish, flax seeds, chia seeds, and walnuts. Despite their presence in many delicious foods, many people lack these essential compounds. The two most important long-chain Omega-3s are eicosapentaenoic acid (EPA) and docosahexaenoic acid (DHA). While both types support brain function, a significant portion of your brain mass is actually made of DHA! (Remember, 81 mg of aspirin can enhance the anti-inflammatory effects of both of these compounds.) A review of the health benefits of omega-3 supplementation suggested that they can help combat the effects of age-related cognitive diseases such as Alzheimer's disease. A review of several studies from the past 15 years indicates that omega-3s can support cognitive function and reduce plaque burden in brains with Alzheimer's disease. A diet rich in omega-3s also reduces the amount of some inflammatory cytokines in patients with Alzheimer's, thus promoting healthy intercellular communication (Vedin et al., 2008).

Because these compounds are abundant in fatty fish, consuming fish oil is the most common supplement method. While many people remember the unpleasant experience of taking cod liver oil in liquid form as children, you can now buy capsules of fish oil that are much easier to swallow! If you're not interested in taking an omega-3 supplement – a tasty alternative would be eating at least eight ounces of seafood a week to help you meet your omega-3 needs. (NIH, 2008)

- **Mitochondria Boosters**

As mitochondrial dysfunction is an important hallmark of aging, it's not surprising that significant efforts have been made to find ways to restore these essential organelles to full function. In this section, we've already looked into a number of supplements that activate the genes of the survival circuit, including AMPK activators, NAD+ boosters, ECGC, and more that work to improve mitochondrial function.

NAC, which stands for *N-acetyl L-cysteine*, is one of the most well-known antioxidants (Pedre et al., 2021), and studies indicate it is a mitochondrial booster. One study establishes NAC as a protective agent against mitochondrial dysfunction, suggesting this occurs because NAC increases levels of the protective compound glutathione in the mitochondria and preserves the process of S-glutathionylation, which protects against oxidative damage (Aparicio-Trejo, 2019). While this study focused on protecting against kidney damage, another study from Baylor College specifically investigated the effects of supplementing with NAC and glycine. Glycine is a common amino acid and chemical precursor to glutathione, an antioxidant comprised of three amino acids, including glycine. Glutathione levels diminish as people age. The Baylor College study showed that these supplements could preserve cognition and muscle strength in older adults while also decreasing bodily inflammation (Baylor College of Medicine, 2021).

Please remember to speak to your doctor about any vitamin regimen you'd like to begin so you can protect yourself and stay safe. Doing your own research is informative, but doctors generally know more about possible drug interactions, allergic reactions, etc., than most of us do. So, always err on the side of caution.

Smart Exercise for Anti-Aging

 "Those who think they have no time for bodily exercise will sooner or later have to find time for illness."

— EDWARD STANLEY

While dietary changes and supplements are a key part of an anti-aging lifestyle, there's much more to combating aging. Another lifestyle intervention that is an essential part of tackling aging is getting enough of the right kind of exercise. From the "We-space" perspective, a nurturing environment (positive support networks, institutions, and businesses that cater to one's exercise objectives) can make a significant difference in attaining your exercise goals and their associated anti-aging benefits.

Modern life is hectic, and many people feel they don't have enough time to exercise. Between work, commuting, cooking, shopping, and time with family, it can become overwhelming to fit exercise into a packed day. Quadrant 1, the quadrant of human existence most concerned with an individual's thoughts and attitudes, has changed drastically over the past 100 years. Modern Western society is one of the most sedentary in history. For many, exercise has become a low priority, something to do if time is left at the end of the day. From a review of literature in the journal *Sports Medicine* on the health benefits of accumulated versus continuous exercise, research suggests that doing a number of short exercise bouts, when you can fit them in, produces similar health benefits as a single but longer bout (Murphy, Blair, and Murtagh, 2009). Therefore, if you don't have the time to complete a full exercise routine, you could cut your normal exercise period in half or even thirds and generally get the same benefits. Knowing this is helpful because you may only exercise if you feel you have the time. In short, short bouts count!

In contrast, people in Blue Zones have daily responsibilities requiring active participation. Therefore, integrating activity into a daily routine is an easy way to increase daily exercise. For instance, taking the stairs instead of the elevator, parking further away in the parking lot from your destination, or adding a 10-minute walk at lunchtime can all help you get more exercise. As we stated, research affirms that short bouts of exercise provide you as much benefit as long bouts, and this was reiterated in an editorial by Emmanuel Stamatakis of the University of Sydney. In addition, short, more intense bouts give you more bang for your buck. For example, there's more exercise benefit to jogging up stairs than walking.

However, sometimes we may not feel supported to exercise by the infrastructure around us. Quadrant 4, the corporate, governmental, and institutional perspective, explains why many of us struggle to get adequate exercise. For example, riding your bike safely in most cities is next to impossible. Walking or jogging in parks by yourself may feel threatening. Your workplace may not offer a workout facility. Private gyms or other workout and exercise facilities can be expensive, time-consuming, and difficult to schedule into your day.

In addition, some people dislike going to the gym because of previous bad experiences, shyness, or because they prefer to exercise outside. While less appealing for nature lovers, there are several benefits to exercising at a gym or in a fitness class with like-minded people who share exercise goals (Quadrant 2 – family/community/cultural influences). Going to the gym or taking a fitness class can facilitate new friendships and a sense of community and foster a sense of belonging and accomplishment. It also encourages people to make a habit of exercising routinely. Again, finding a class, workout partner, or group gives you "cultural" support and makes exercise easier to sustain for many.

Exercise, in general, is an essential aspect of an anti-aging lifestyle for two reasons: Not only does it promote longevity, but it also keeps you strong and able so you can fully enjoy the extra years you get as a result. A fascinating 2018 study showed that women who were sedentary in their middle age were more likely to experience dementia in their senior years than women who were physically fit in middle age. Of the women that did develop dementia, those who were sedentary in their middle age developed dementia much earlier than their active counterparts—11 years earlier on average (American Academy of Neurology, 2018). Men's brains can also benefit from physical fitness. A co-ed 2017 study showed that early-stage Alzheimer's patients who performed regular aerobic exercises improved their physical fitness at the end of the 26-week experiment and retained more of their daily functioning and memory recall than those who performed non-aerobic exercises (Morris et al., 2017).

Recall the idea of *hormesis* or "good stress" discussed in the previous chapter. That is, a measure of stress causes epigenetic changes to help the body weather the situation. Hormesis activates a number of genes associated with survival and resilience, leading to a reduction in oxidative stress and a boost in mitochondrial function (Ji, Gomez-Cabera, and Vina, 2006). Not only that, but exercise can also reduce bodily inflammation, which is responsible for many of the health problems we associate with aging. For example, one review showed that exercise decreases inflammation and the risk of high blood pressure and related disease. The positive effects of exercise on the gut microbiome could also contribute to these health benefits (Chen et al., 2018). While endless forms of exercise can benefit your health, not every type of exercise is created equal, and some will support your anti-aging goals more than others.

Before going into the types of exercise that are most beneficial from an anti-aging perspective, it's worth mentioning that you should consult your doctor before starting any new exercise routine, especially if you have preexisting health problems.

Interval Training

Performing enough continuous and repetitive work during exercise to achieve hormesis is difficult. Most people who attempt to exercise this way do not achieve hormesis because of the time it requires. Therefore, people don't feel or see much change and end up bored and frustrated. Consequently, many may quit their exercise routine.

Interval training addresses these issues:

1. It includes short bouts of exercise intense enough to achieve hormesis. Because of its limited duration, it feels less daunting for most people.
2. It usually includes a variety of exercises, so there is less chance of boredom.
3. Rest periods allow people to recuperate between bouts of intense exercise.

Though the intensity of exercise may vary based on age, level of fitness, etc., regardless, a relatively high level of intensity across the board is necessary to achieve hormesis.

The most well-known cardiovascular (cardio) type of interval workout is High-Intensity Interval Training (HIIT). Basic interval training improves your speed, agility, and cardiovascular fitness. A person with good cardio fitness can usually work out longer and more intensely without getting out of breath. While interval training is extremely popular with runners, swimmers, track and field athletes, and others who participate in sports that demand high cardio activity, almost anyone looking to improve their cardio fitness can benefit from this kind of training.

There is scientific backing to support the idea that interval training is an efficient and effective way to achieve cardiovascular health. For example, a study by Phillips et al. in 2017 suggests that it's challenging for many adults to reach the recommended amount of cardio activity per week (roughly 150 minutes). However, interval training can help because it intensifies the work effort enough that the overall duration of the workout can be shorter.

Another type of interval training involves using weights, or body weight, to benefit the musculoskeletal and cardiovascular systems. A study was conducted on male and female volunteers who showed signs of insulin resistance or type II diabetes. The researchers found that the volunteers who participated in interval training exhibited lower mean blood pressure and fasting insulin resistance at the end of the study (Phillips et al., 2017). Recalling that deregulated nutrient sensing (like insulin resistance) and poor cardiac health are common health problems associated with aging, this study suggests that interval training can be an important part of an anti-aging exercise routine.

Strength Training

While many think strength training only refers to weightlifting, this term actually covers a broad range of exercises. Any exercise that uses *resistance,* or a piece of equipment that requires physical strength to move, falls under the purview of strength training. Some examples are free weights such as dumbbells and barbells, weight and pulley machines, resistance bands, and medicine balls. And as mentioned earlier, you can even perform strength training exercises using your body weight, such as push-ups, squats, and even yoga poses.

Strength training focuses on the musculoskeletal system that facilitates your body's movement. The three key reasons for strength training are strengthening muscles and bones, increasing mobility, and improving overall health. Working against resistance through strength training creates minuscule tears in muscle tissue that subsequently rebuild, making them stronger. Also, studies have shown that muscles pulling on bones during strength training make bones stronger (Gomez-Cabello et al., 2012). Using these training methods to stress muscles and bones to strengthen them is yet another example of hormesis at work. Strength training can be done to target specific muscles, allowing you to work out one group of muscles one day and another group the next day, giving the first group a chance to rest and rebuild. Of course, performing strength training with proper form and awareness of your abilities is critical to prevent injury. Still, it can significantly boost your daily functioning and general health when done correctly. For example, another study suggests that strength training improves the strength and durability of your entire body structure—not just the skeletal muscles and bones but also joints, tendons, and ligaments (Fleck and Falkel, 1986). These benefits are important to older adults who are at risk of becoming frail and can help to reduce their risk of injury from falls. Older adults tend to undergo a decrease in muscle mass as they age, and the promotion of muscle protein synthesis through strength training can help combat this process (Aguirre and Villareal, 2015). The same review by Aguirre and Villareal showed a general increase in functioning in adults over 65 who underwent combined resistance and aerobic training.

Strength training also increases metabolism and combats mitochondrial dysfunction. For example, one study on post-menopausal women showed higher mitochondrial volumes and larger mitochondria after 12 months of regular strength training (Manfredi et al., 2014).

Yoga and Stretching

Many older adults struggle with balance and flexibility as they age, making it harder to enjoy physical activity and increasing their risk for injury when performing daily tasks. One way to combat this is to include yoga or stretching in your daily exercise routine. Stretching engages muscles and also involves connective tissue, including fascia and ligaments, which link muscles, bones, blood vessels, and organs in your body. Any stretching exercise extends and flexes specific muscles, improving range of motion and strengthening those muscles. Standing stretches involve fine muscle control, which may help improve balance, minimizing the potential for falls. In particular, Dr. Jinsup Song of the Gait Institute conducted a study with 24 older women that seems to support this (Song, 2008).

Stretching can also be used to alleviate muscle cramps. But, again, this isn't just for older adults. Athletes in virtually every sport stretch before and after workouts and, in many cases, throughout the day.

Yoga is a very ancient form of exercise that incorporates stretching techniques. The practitioner moves through a series of prescribed positions that help to improve strength, balance, and flexibility. Controlled breathing and meditative techniques are also a part of some forms of yoga. The practice of yoga originated in India, and its original purpose was to help the practitioner achieve a spiritual state of tranquility. However, it has spread worldwide and is now popular with people of all cultures and faiths. Many people who dislike stretching enjoy yoga and reap numerous benefits. For example, a study of a group of volunteers who practiced yoga and meditation for 12 weeks had lower biochemical markers of aging and higher markers associated with longevity (such as SIRT1) in comparison to a control group of the same age (Tolahunase, Sagar, and Dada, 2017). Additionally, one review that explored the effects of yoga on age-related health problems suggested that yoga could reduce the severity of neurodegenerative illnesses by countering depression, anxiety, and stress, as well as reducing memory loss. It also suggests that yoga could help reduce oxidative stress on the body, reducing age-related DNA damage and, thus, genomic instability (Mohammed et al., 2018).

Whether you learn to practice yoga or an alternate type of stretching, keeping safety in mind is essential. Knowing your physical strength and abilities is important when deciding whether to perform a new stretching exercise or yoga pose. For example, trying a yoga pose without the strength and balance to maintain it can lead to a fall. In addition, improper stretching can damage the tendons, ligaments, and muscle fibers. Therefore, practicing proper alignment and biomechanics is essential to avoid injury. Attending a group fitness class can be beneficial; this way, an instructor can guide you as you learn how to stretch. If you do not have access to yoga or stretching classes in your immediate area (a Quadrant 4 issue – corporate, governmental, or institutional limitation), you might want to avail yourself of yoga or stretching classes taught through online portals, such as the free option of YouTube (Quadrant 4 – corporate, governmental, or institutional alternative).

Our Exercise Routine

Based on this research, we designed an exercise routine for ourselves that we supplement with regular walks. It consists of: a 5-minute cardiovascular warm-up (walking or jogging) to warm muscles. Then 20 minutes of interval training using strength and resistance equipment or body weight for short intervals (1–2 minutes) followed by a period of rest (30 seconds–1 ½ minutes). Our session concludes with 5 minutes of full-body yoga or stretching. This three-pronged approach combines the benefits of strength and resistance training, a cardiovascular workout derived from the intensity of the intervals, and stretching. We feel it allows us to garner the most benefits in a relatively short period of time.

Exercise and the Gut Microbiome

Surprisingly, exercise also has a highly beneficial effect on your gut microbiome. Scientists are learning more every year about how the systems that keep our bodies running are intertwined, leading to a tsunami of research into the previously unknown effects of the gut microbiome on the rest of our bodies and vice versa. Recent research on the gut microbiome and exercise shows that the benefits of exercise impact more than just your musculoskeletal and cardiovascular systems. Generally, people who exercise regularly *and* eat a healthy diet to support their physical health have greater gut biodiversity and more beneficial species than the average person.

In *Gut Crisis*, Wallace references a 2014 study comparing the gut microbiota of professional athletes with those of people who were generally sedentary, like most individuals in Western society. The results of the study were fascinating. Generally, the athletes who volunteered for the project had a much more diverse gut microbiome than sedentary people. The researchers noted that the athlete's microbiome contained a higher level of a beneficial species of gut bacteria known as *Akkermansia muciniphilla* than the control group. This species of bacteria is found in much lower quantities in people who are obese or dealing with other metabolic issues like insulin resistance. Of course, it's impossible to discount the effects of diet when interpreting this study's findings because professional athletes typically eat a diet higher in protein than the average person. Rather than cite exercise as the main cause of the difference between the groups' gut microbiomes, the researchers suggested that the high-protein diet consumed by athletes also influenced the increased gut biodiversity and associated benefits (Clarke et al., 2014).

Another example of the benefits of a physically active lifestyle is examined in a scientific review which shows the relationship between exercise, cardiac health, and the gut microbiome. The review concluded that exercise positively affects cardiac health, specifically "hyperlipidemia, hypertension, abdominal obesity, diabetes, and psychosocial factors" (Chen et al., 2014). This study also suggests that physically active people had more diverse gut microbiomes with higher populations of beneficial species and lower populations of some harmful species (Chen et al., 2014).

Healthy Mind, Healthy Body

Exercise and diet aren't the only aspects of a healthy lifestyle. Taking care of your mental and emotional health is essential to your overall well-being. Quadrant 2 (family/community/cultural influences) suggests that our mental and emotional health is influenced by the communities in which we live, positively or negatively. For example, you may enjoy the atmosphere of sitting at the beach and spending time with friends but dislike traffic and crowds. In other words, your mental and emotional health does not exist in a vacuum. The book *The Blue Zones* suggests that in areas of the world where people live the longest, the quality of mental and emotional health is positively influenced by their local communities. For example, in many Blue Zones, elders have an intrinsic sense of purpose during that stage of their lives. By contrast, people in Western societies may feel a lack of purpose or meaning in their senior years, especially if they've retired. This cultural difference suggests that people in Western society should seriously consider the nature of the community in which they live to be sure it supports their mental and emotional well-being.

In particular, to promote long life and health spans, you may need to take matters into your own hands (Quadrant 1 – personal beliefs/understandings/experiences) and evaluate whether or not you live in a culture that supports your mental and emotional well-being. Here are some questions to consider: Would living with like-minded folks enhance your mental and emotional health, or would diversity be more to your liking? Would you rather live with people of the same faith, ethnicity, culture, age, gender, political orientation, etc.? You might want to assess answers to these questions in the framework of the Quadrants. That is, reflect on your desires and needs (Q1), assess what kind of culture nurtures those needs and wants (Q2), consider if your culture supports scientific research and its application to health (Q3), and evaluate if there are corporations, institutions, and governmental entities in your community that support health and well-being, (e.g., hospitals, health clubs, parks and recreation) (Q4).

Meditation and Pranayama

 "Meditation is a vital way to purify and quiet the mind, thus rejuvenating the body."

— DEEPAK CHOPRA

There are many different meditation and pranayama (breath work) practices. Some have been scientifically tested for their effects on physiology, while the efficacy of others relies on personal experiences. Either way, people meditate or practice pranayama for many different reasons. Though meditation and pranayama involve a time commitment and discipline, science and experience suggest they offer mental and emotional health benefits.

First, we'll focus on the benefits of meditation. Depending on the meditation type and practitioner's intent, a person could gain spiritual insight, achieve a state of tranquility, or learn to let go of the stressful things in their life. Others may seek to develop positive traits such as patience, compassion, and forgiveness or build internal spiritual energy—these are just a few examples. Meditation can be performed while sitting, lying down, standing, or walking for a short or long time, with or without ritual objects such as prayer beads, a lit candle, etc. In addition, many people burn incense or listen to calming music or tones while meditating.

Scientific evidence shows meditation can help quell mental health issues like anxiety and depression. Additionally, meditation can have physiological and biological effects, like reducing blood pressure and inducing anti-aging genes. For example, one study on the impact of yoga and meditation on cellular aging indicated that these practices help generate SIRT-1 and other beneficial compounds. This same study also showed reduced levels of the stress hormone cortisol and *8-hydroxy-2'-deoxyguanosine* (8-OH2dG). This is good news because high levels of these two markers signal DNA damage and indicate genomic instability, thereby promoting aging (Tolahunase, Sagar, and Dana, 2017). Just like with exercise, not every form of meditation is created equal, and some may be more helpful to those following anti-aging lifestyles than others. One form of meditation with significant scientific evidence to support its benefits is Transcendental Meditation (TM), which uses a mantra to "naturally and effortlessly" quiet the mind (Scientific Research on Maharishi's Transcendental Meditation and TM-Sidhi Programme: Collected Papers, Volumes 1- 8). This technique allows practitioners to experience a state of "deep rest," physiologically twice as deep as the deepest sleep. This is important as it gives the body a deep rejuvenating rest, releasing physical and emotional stress and consequently improving the practitioner's overall health. Ample scientific research suggests that TM benefits a practitioner's physical, mental, and emotional health.

One study measured TM practitioners' "biological age" compared to the general public. Biological age is different from a person's chronological age. Biological age measures a person's physical decline due to age, genetics, lifestyle, and disease using a range of physical biomarkers. The study found that practitioners of TM had, on average, a biological age 5-12 years younger than those in the general population, depending on how long they had been practicing (Wallace et al., 1981). Finally, there is also data to suggest that TM can reduce inflammation (Klemons, 1972), combating several hallmarks of aging.

Many schools of meditation involve breath control, and controlling one's breathing can, in and of itself, be a beneficial lifestyle choice. An extensive review of the health benefits of breath control practices showed distinct physiological changes. One parameter this review examined is heart rate variability (HRV), which is precisely what it sounds like: a measure of how variable, on average, the length of time is between heartbeats. A high HRV indicates a relaxed person, while a low HRV indicates the person is under stress. The review indicated that practicing breath control, which temporarily stresses your body (another form of hormesis), lowers HRV. However, when the body recovers from the stress, the HRV increases, signaling that the body was able to return to a restful state yet is now better prepared for future stresses (Zaccaro et al., 2018). However, remember that chronic stress is not good as it is associated with many age-related diseases, including heart disease and type II diabetes.

One of the significant types of breath control that this review examined is *pranayama*, a very ancient practice originating from Hinduism. Pranayama, which translates to both "the stop/control" and "rising/expansion of breath" in the original Sanskrit, was originally a part of the practice of yoga. Others describe *prana* as "life force" and Yama as a "bridle" or "rein." Pranayama, like TM, has been shown to have clear health benefits, especially in regard to aging, like reducing genomic instability and slowing telomere attrition (Zaccaro et al., 2018). Pranayama, together with asana, also appears to be able to reduce genomic instability and slow telomere attrition (*Asana* is a Vedic term defined as "seat" by ancient Vedic scriptures, modern-day asanas are both seated and standing poses, usually moving from one to the next). The researchers propose that the breathing technique accomplishes this by increasing the amount of oxygen reaching the body's cells (Rathore and Abraham, 2018).

Community, Religiosity, and Sense of Purpose

> *"We don't stop playing because we grow old; we grow old because we stop playing."*

> — GEORGE BERNARD SHAW

When writing this book, I, John, recalled how people I knew seemed to live longer or shorter depending on their respective outlooks on life. Those family or friends who maintained a passion for living in their later years took care of themselves, stayed active and engaged, seemed to enjoy their lives more, and tended to live longer. Conversely, those family or friends who perceived their later years as an inevitable downhill slide to ill health and loneliness seemed to pass away relatively early with more emotional and physical suffering.

Based on these personal reflections, we did some research and found evidence showing that retirement itself can adversely influence longevity. One study revealed that about 40% of retired participants were more likely to suffer a heart attack or stroke than participants who decided to continue working (Skerrett, 2012). This had me reflect on a boss I knew who retired relatively early but then passed away within six months of retirement. This personal experience is consistent with the above study that found ill health effects were more pronounced in the first year of retirement, after which things leveled off. This same study did acknowledge that other studies reveal that retirees' health can improve. Yet, other studies showed no measurable differences in health between those who retired and those who continued to work. This variation in study findings suggests that it may depend on your job before you retired, what you decided to do after retirement, and, if you have one, how healthy your spousal relationship is at retirement. For example, suppose you had a passion for your job and enjoyed the social network it provided. In that case, retirement might have you feeling alone and uninspired, lacking the motivation to engage in new ventures. If you feel isolated, you may feel time passing quickly and become depressed, especially if you don't stay active and challenge yourself.

On the other hand, if you hated your job and it stressed you out, you might find retirement an emotional and physical relief. You might engage in fun and exciting activities you previously didn't have time for, finding your health and relationships improving over time. As Ken Wilber would suggest, your perspective on life could make all the difference and determine whether or not you thrive in your retirement years.

Another personal example of how things could go differently in our older years was highlighted by the difference between my maternal and paternal grandmothers— both of whom I loved dearly. My paternal grandmother led an active and engaging life in her later years, becoming the head of a tenant advocacy group at her retirement home. She lived to a healthy, ripe old age. Yet, my maternal grandmother seemed to "get along" each day (just surviving), alone in her home and requiring support from family. Eventually, she was moved to a high-care convalescent home, where she died after several years of mental and physical suffering. Another more shocking example I will never forget was shared by a man in my prostate cancer support group who confessed he didn't want to pursue cancer treatment (for this relatively treatable cancer).

The man explained that he saw his kids become successful adults with their own families. He believed that his job as a father was complete, and he could now accept his cancer diagnosis and leave this world in peace. Every man in the group was stunned, and many reached out to him after the session to encourage him to change his attitude because there was so much to look forward to in his life, especially moments with his grandkids. Unfortunately, we never learned of the man's fate, as he didn't return to any more meetings.

Though these personal stories are anecdotal, research supports the notion that being socially active and maintaining personal goals could positively affect the quality and longevity of our lives. It made us stop and think that we have the power to positively influence our longevity by taking care of ourselves, maintaining a positive attitude, staying engaged in life, and setting challenging personal goals that promote physical, emotional, and intellectual growth.

As we have already mentioned, Quadrant 2 (family/community/cultural influences) and Quadrant 4 (corporate/governmental/institutional influences) suggest how having a like-minded community around us can have an incredible effect on our thoughts and choices (Quadrant 1 – personal beliefs/understandings/experiences). Therefore, surrounding ourselves with like-minded people who practice a healthy, anti-aging lifestyle can make it easier for us to adopt and sustain healthy anti-aging behaviors.

In fact, for some of the longest-lived people in the world, the healthy behaviors we consider revolutionary anti-aging lifestyle changes are simply a normal way of life. For example, Dan Buettner, author of *The Blue Zones*, has made a career out of researching the cultures and habits of the world's longest-lived communities to discover what the basis of their extraordinarily long lifespans could be. He discusses several communities in rural Sardinia, a region of Italy known for its high life expectancy. As a case in point, he notes that most families in rural Sardinian communities make their living as farmers or shepherds. The average Sardinian shepherd burns 490 calories an hour walking up and down the region's steep slopes (Buettner, 2017). To equal this, one would have to walk briskly for two hours a day—a radical lifestyle change for most North Americans but a typical routine for many in Sardinia!

Not only can the people around you profoundly affect your beliefs, daily practices, and sense of "normal," but they can also have a physiological effect by influencing your microbiome. In *The Longevity Paradox*, Gundry suggests that the people around you can directly affect which bacteria are most present in your microbiome, stating, "People who are not genetically related but live in the same household have strikingly similar gut microbiomes" as a result of sharing the same space, habits, and routines (Gundry, 2019). Further, another study suggests that gut bacteria directly affect the quality of your health. In this study, researchers used pairs of identical twins, one thin and one obese. Fecal samples were collected from the respective volunteers and then transplanted into mice that were lab-engineered to be born without gut microbiota. Essentially, the mice would only have transplanted gut bacteria from one of the twins. Lo and behold, the mice who received "obese" fecal transplants gained weight, while those that received "thin" fecal transplants lost weight. These results suggest that gut bacteria play more of a role in your weight than previously thought (Ridaura et al., 2013). On a practical level, if this is true for humans, weight loss may depend not just on how you eat but also on the people whose bacteria you "share."

Additionally, your microbiota could influence your vulnerability to diseases. For example, if you transplant fecal matter from a person with a healthy microbiome into someone with Irritable Bowel Syndrome (IBS), the person with IBS will show improvements (Vermeire et al., 2016). These are just a few examples that show how vital your microbiome is to your health.

All things considered, the people in your life can affect your health in ways you may never have dreamed of. So, it's worth considering whether your family, friends, and community (Quadrant 2 – family/community/cultural influences) support your health goals. Suppose the people around you do not support you in making changes to improve your health. In that case, it's worth considering whether they're the people you want to spend time with (a Quadrant 1 decision – personal beliefs/understandings/experiences). Looking for a new social group, changing jobs, or even relocating entirely are all things to consider if you find yourself in an unsupportive environment.

Your social circle isn't the only place where it's important to receive support for healthy lifestyle changes. It's also crucial that your medical provider (Quadrant 4 – corporate/governmental/institutional influences) is supportive and open-minded. Some doctors are open to anti-aging life-style choices, especially those practicing functional or integrative medicine which focuses on a holistic approach to health.

While religion and spirituality have recently declined in popularity in some regions, being part of a religious or spiritual community (Quadrant 4 – corporate/governmental/institutional influences) can be beneficial. Looking back at the different Levels of Development, almost all of them, except for Beige (Archaic-Instinctual) and Orange (Scientific Achievement), include spirituality as a factor. For example, in *The Blue Zones*, many of the centenarians interviewed were active in some kind of religious community. Belonging to a group of like-minded people provides a person with a source of positivity, reducing chronic stress that drives inflammation, a significant marker of aging. Not only that, but religious or spiritual beliefs can give a person an essential sense of purpose and provide them with a community that potentially supports their health choices (Buettner, 2017).

In *The Blue Zones*, Buettner describes how older adults in Blue Zone communities have a strong sense of purpose. They play an integral role in the family unit, which motivates them to stay active and optimistic into their old age. In this way, an older person is welcomed into meaningful participation in life that supports them in having a full, productive, and healthy lifespan. In one anecdote, Buettner describes how all the centenarians told him that their families were the most important thing in their world, sometimes even describing family as their purpose in life. They lived with or near their children and grandchildren, who cared for them into their old age (Buettner, 2017). On the flip side, in North America, many older people live apart from their families and consequently may lack a strong sense of purpose through their connection with family. However, if a strong sense of purpose and connection leads to longer and happier lives, it would be wise for older adults to take the initiative to cultivate a strong relationship with their extended family. This investment also puts long-term care front and center for family members of older adults, destined to decline as they age. If direct family involvement is not possible or practical, there are other ways to develop a sense of purpose and belonging. Alternatives could include internet interactions with family and friends or joining like-minded individuals in purposeful activities like volunteering in community child care and pet care programs.

WHY DOES IT MATTER?

Throughout this book, we've looked at how each Quadrant of Human Existence presents information about longevity and aging. In addition, we've touched on how a person's Level of Development affects how they process information about aging and their likelihood to make anti-aging lifestyle changes. Finally, we've discussed several ways to incorporate anti-aging practices into one's daily health routine.

There's more to an anti-aging lifestyle than just taking the right supplements. Making the change to an anti-aging lifestyle can be a lot of work and requires personal accountability and some level of sacrifice. In most cases, people will have to decide whether the upsides of an anti-aging lifestyle outweigh the downsides. Unfortunately, few are fully aware of the pros and cons of the typical Western or anti-aging lifestyles to make informed decisions. For example, many people are unaware of the health consequences of eating wheat gluten and lectins or having an unhealthy gut microbiome. Furthermore, while it's more well-known that sugar, red meat, and saturated fats are unhealthy, many people eat them out of convenience, habit, or because they feel the experience is worth the risks— that is until they experience their first heart attack!

In the last few chapters, we've seen that improving your diet, taking supplements, adopting an efficient exercise routine, looking into spiritual practices or meditation, and finding a positive community are all important aspects of an anti-aging lifestyle. For most people, making all these changes will take some time, as old habits die hard, and trying to change your life too drastically or too quickly can set you up for a backslide. Every level of development has something to offer, and moving through each one is a stepping stone to the next level of growth. Just like that old metaphor about learning to crawl before you can walk, take it step by step. Personal accountability around health, wellness, and pursuing a long and healthy lifespan is key. Each choice you make is important, but equally important is to refrain from beating yourself up if you make a poor choice occasionally! Don't be victimized by yourself or others. Plenty of resources are available to assist you in achieving your anti-aging goals by helping you make healthy and responsible choices.

PART IV: THE FUTURE OF ANTI-AGING

U p to this point, we've looked deeply into what kinds of anti-aging interventions are accessible right now, ranging from diets to supplements to exercising and meditation. But now that more research on aging and how we can combat it is taking place, doors are being opened to new interventions that were previously unavailable. This chapter will close out our book by briefly examining the medical interventions for aging that may be available in the coming years or decades. Please don't take the promising information in this chapter as a reason not to adopt healthier lifestyle behaviors now. Switching up your diet and making other anti-aging lifestyle changes can help increase the odds that you'll be around to take full advantage of these and other upcoming interventions as they become available!

STEM CELL THERAPY

Stem cell therapy is a controversial topic in many circles, primarily due to ethical concerns surrounding the use of embryonic stem cells. However, stem cell therapies are among the most promising anti-aging medical interventions currently being investigated, and forms of stem cell therapy are already in use.

As you know, stem cells are undifferentiated cells that our bodies use to replenish cell populations that can't replenish by dividing. They are also used to repair damaged or injured organs or tissues. As stem cells can differentiate into a wide range of cell types, there's great medical interest in using them to cure various and previously untreatable issues. For example, stem cell exhaustion is a primary hallmark of aging that plays a role in the increasing frailty and declining immune systems from which many older people suffer. Finding ways to replenish stem cells or to deliver them to areas of the body that aren't ordinarily accessible would make it possible to repair age-related damage previously thought to be irreversible. Some forms of stem cell therapy are already used to treat everything from arthritis to Alzheimer's, but we'll likely see even more advancements in the future (Sinclair, 2019).

Shinya Yamanaka, a stem cell researcher and Nobel Prize recipient in 2012, was responsible for discovering a combination of four genes that, if activated, could induce differentiated adult cells to revert to immature pluripotent stem cells. Like regular stem cells, these could differentiate into any other kind of cell (Okita, Ichisaka, and Yamanaka, 2007). This discovery means that patients could harvest their own already differentiated adult cells and turn them into stem cells that are a perfect biological match. Consequently, they could be used to grow needed tissues or even organs that their bodies and immune systems would not reject. The method also reduces ethical concerns around the use of embryonic stem cells. The possibilities for technologies based on Yamanaka's discovery are being explored by his and other laboratories, with very promising results. A good example is a 2016 trial where stem cells were effective in reversing age-related vision loss in a 78-year-old woman (Foundation Fighting Blindness, 2016). This type of stem cell research offers a hopeful future for people suffering from challenging age-related diseases.

DNA REPROGRAMMING

The phrase "DNA reprogramming" sounds like something out of science fiction, but actually, this is a promising avenue for future anti-aging interventions! Of course, the safety and efficacy of gene therapy treatments are still being investigated, and most of them have yet to be approved for widespread use. Still, early forms of this technology show great promise in tackling aging at its root.

While there are different proposed methods of reprogramming human and animal DNA in living adults, a promising one uses adenoviruses, a type of virus that inserts its genome into the DNA molecule of a host cell. A form of gene therapy using adenoviruses can cure blindness caused by a mutation in the RPE65 gene. A virus containing the gene is inserted into the patient's retina, which quickly proliferates and delivers the gene to the cells in the eye (Utz et al., 2019). Since eyes are immunologically isolated from the rest of the body, the virus couldn't spread further. In *Lifespan*, Sinclair expresses hope this technology will eventually be used to insert additional copies of longevity-associated genes (possibly the Yamanaka factors) into the rest of the body to create a therapy that reverses all hallmarks of aging in one treatment (Sinclair, 2019).

CATALYTIC ANTIBODIES

The SENS Foundation (Strategies for Engineered Negligible Senescence) is an organization that funds research into anti-aging medical interventions. While SENS is currently reporting on a wide range of fascinating studies, one that stands out is an antibody therapy known as Aducanumab, or Aduhelm, which has recently completed Phase III clinical trials and is now being tried out as a treatment for Alzheimer's disease in some hospitals (SENS, 2021). Aducanumab targets extracellular protein aggregates linked to the development of Alzheimer's disease in the brain. While these aggregates form quickly in the brains of patients with Alzheimer's, they can also develop in other tissues, causing inflammation and impairing organ function.

To clear these aggregates out of the body and prevent the loss of organ function, Aducanumab uses specialized antibodies that bind to aggregates, marking them for removal from the tissue by the immune system. While these antibodies can be produced out of the body and intravenously infused, the human body can also be trained to make them in-house. Activating these antibodies is done by injecting the patient with fragments of the amyloids or with mRNAs that code for the unwanted proteins, using similar technologies to vaccination (SENS, 2021).

This technology has been further developed by the laboratory of Dr. Sudhir Paul, who conducted his research at Texas-Houston Medical School. Rather than rely on regular anti-bodies to clear aggregates, which can cause inflammation and also deplete the antibodies over time, Paul's version of the treatment depends on *catabodies*, which are antibodies that destroy bound protein aggregates without relying on the rest of the immune system and without destroying themselves in the process. The researchers envision that this technology will be used to create "longevity vaccines" that prevent age-related amyloid buildup throughout the body before it starts (Planque, Massey, and Paul, 2020).

BIOMARKERS AND METRICS

Biological markers, better known as biomarkers, are measurable characteristics of a biological state. They can indicate normal or healthy functioning, abnormal or unhealthy functioning, or responses to treatments and therapies. Metrics is a term for measuring or quantifying something, such as biological markers.

Quantifying allows for comparing and contrasting data from different individuals and can, with enough data, support establishing norms as well as revealing anomalies. A common biomarker is measuring one's temperature. The established norm for an individual's healthy temperature is represented at

98.6 degrees. However, some people may have a "normal" temperature a little above or below this metric, but too much of a discrepancy likely indicates some disease state. Over time, research on various diseases, causes of death, cancers, etc., has expanded the number and kind of biomarkers doctors can monitor. Here is a list of common, existing biomarkers that can be used by your doctor (if not already used) to gauge your current state of health, as well as your progress toward improving your health, wellness, youthfulness, and longevity:

- Blood pressure
- Body fat levels
- Hormone levels
- Auditory and visual thresholds
- Immune function
- Temperature regulation
- Bone density
- Muscle strength
- Skin thickness
- Cholesterol levels
- Blood sugar tolerance
- Lung capacity
- Mental capacity
- Flexibility

As anti-aging research intensifies, it is almost inevitable that additional biomarkers and ways to measure them will be found. Such indicators might include ways to quantify our gut microbiome diversity, additional hormone markers, expanded blood markers, advanced genetic testing, and telomere attrition.

These measures will not only allow better disease diagnoses but also allow doctors to uncover unhealthy situations much earlier so interventions can be employed sooner. In addition, the future of biomarking may advance ways of preventing a potential disease from manifesting in the first place. Monitoring biomarkers (for overall health and longevity) will become more personal and "real-time" as devices are developed for us to wear or implant under our skin so that they can alert us of unhealthy situations more quickly, like today's blood sugar monitors for people with diabetes. Someday, car seats could be engineered to indicate if your heartbeat is irregular, alert authorities for timely intervention, and possibly prevent an accident. Computer keyboards could be designed to show signs of Parkinson's Disease or Multiple Sclerosis based on an individual's keystrokes. Given the possibilities of future research, scientific discoveries, real-time biomonitoring, and subsequent preventive measures and interventions, is it hard to imagine we could achieve a reality of effectively reversing aging and prolonging a healthy life?

SHARE THE KNOWLEDGE

You'll notice an incredible difference when you start making these changes, which puts you in the perfect position to help other people like you.

Simply by sharing your honest opinion of this book and a little about your own experience, you'll show new readers that they too can reverse the effects of aging – and you'll show them exactly where they can find the guidance that will help them get there.

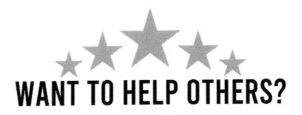

WANT TO HELP OTHERS?

Thank you for your support. We're excited about the future ahead of you.

Scan the QR code below for a quick review!

CONCLUSION

 "And in the end, it's not the years in your life that count. It's the life in your years."

— ABRAHAM LINCOLN

Throughout this book, we've touched on the physical and psychological aspects of aging and the anti-aging movement, ranging from the physical effects of aging to the methods available to combat it. We've also looked at the impact of society's assumptions about aging and how we can turn our mindsets around to open up the possibility of a brighter, healthier, and longer future.

Though the improvements in our own lives are anecdotal, they result from lifestyle changes based on our understanding of the anti-aging research we've read. Here are some improvements we've noticed in our personal health beyond what we've already mentioned: We have seen age spots on our skin start to fade, and the quality of our skin has become less dry and more supple. Meditation lowered John's blood pressure (130/80 in April 2021 to 118/76 in July 2022). John has noticed that he no longer sees any hair in the shower drain, and I, Lisa, have seen my hair get thicker and darker. I'm losing the gray hairs that have been creeping in! Now, my hair is a medium-colored dishwater blonde again, and I'm not sure what to do with it (I used to get my hair highlighted, so maybe I'll have to go back)!

As we iterated earlier in this book, our society is due for a major paradigm shift regarding anti-aging beliefs. The current research points to a revolutionary idea: That aging is a disease that can be combatted like any other, resulting in longer and healthier lifespans for those who choose a healthy anti-aging lifestyle and cutting-edge interventions. While scientific knowledge of how to slow the progress of aging is growing every day, an even more revolutionary idea is emerging. If we can slow the progress of aging, one day, we may be able to stop or even reverse it, at least for a time. Turning back the hands of time may sound like the stuff of science fiction. Still, we hope that our vision of longer, healthier lives becoming more widespread will motivate readers to shift their paradigm on aging and consider what might be possible with new scientific breakthroughs.

An effective approach to an anti-aging lifestyle starts with a thorough understanding of our own level of personal development and recognizing how we are influenced by the four quadrants from which we gather information. This awareness is a predicate for an open mindset, which allows one to assess all sources of information and influence to advance a long, healthy, and productive life. In this book, we have suggested anti-aging practices and behaviors, including a modified diet, supplements, effective exercise, meditation, and social support. Our wish for our readers is that they will feel inspired and motivated to make changes to improve their health and enjoy a long and enhanced health span as a result. *Carpe diem!*

REFERENCES AND NOTES

Abraham, J., & Rathore, M. (2018). Implication of asana, pranayama and meditation on telomere stability. *International Journal of Yoga, 11*(3), 186. https://doi.org/10.4103/ijoy.ijoy_51_17

Aida J., Kondo K., Hirai H., Subramanian S. V., Murata C., Kondo N., et al. Assessing the association between all-cause mortality and multiple aspects of individual social capital among the older Japanese. BMC Public Health. 2011;11:499.

Anderson, R. A., Zhan, Z., Luo, R., Guo, X., Guo, Q., Zhou, J., Kong, J., Davis, P. A., & Stoecker, B. J. (2016). Cinnamon extract lowers glucose, insulin and cholesterol in people with elevated serum glucose. *Journal of Traditional and Complementary Medicine, 6*(4), 332–336. https://doi.org/10.1016/j.jtcme.2015.03.005

Aguirre, L. E., & Villareal, D. T. (2019). Physical exercise as therapy for frailty. *Nestlé Nutrition Institute Workshop Series*, 83–92. https://doi.org/10.1159/000382065

Ahmed, H., Abushouk, A. I., Gabr, M., Negida, A., & Abdel-Daim, M. M. (2017). Parkinson's disease and pesticides: A meta-analysis of disease connection and genetic alterations. *Biomedicine & Pharmacotherapy, 90*, 638–649. https://doi.org/10.1016/j.biopha.2017.03.100

Albertsson, P.-Å., Köhnke, R., Emek, Sinan C., Mei, J., Rehfeld, Jens F., Åkerlund, H.-E., & Erlanson-Albertsson, C. (2007). Chloroplast membranes retard fat digestion and induce satiety: effect of biological membranes on pancreatic lipase/co-lipase. *Biochemical Journal, 401*(3), 727–733. https://doi.org/10.1042/bj20061463

Alliance for Aging Research. (2021). *Home.* Alliance for Aging Research. https://www.agingresearch.org/

American Academy of Neurology. (2018). *Physically fit women nearly 90 percent less likely to develop dementia.* ScienceDaily. https://www.sciencedaily.com/releases/2018/03/180315101805.htm

American Heart Association. (2017, March 23). *Trans fats.* Heart.org. https://www.heart.org/en/healthy-living/healthy-eating/eat-smart/fats/trans-fat

Akbaraly, T. N., Arnaud, J., Rayman, M. P., Hininger-Favier, I., Roussel, A.-M.,

Berr, C., & Fontbonne, A. (2010). Plasma selenium and risk of dysglycemia in an elderly French population: Results from the prospective epidemiology of vascular ageing study. *Nutrition & Metabolism, 7,* 21. https://doi.org/10.1186/1743-7075-7-21

Baglietto-Vargas D, et al. Generation of a humanized Aβ expressing mouse demonstrating aspects of Alzheimer's disease-like pathology. *Nature Communications.* 2021;12(1):2421. https://doi.org/10.1038/s41467-021-22624-z

Baur, J. A., & Sinclair, D. A. (2006). Therapeutic potential of resveratrol: the in vivo evidence. *Nature Reviews. Drug Discovery, 5*(6), 493–506. https://doi.org/10.1038/nrd2060

Baylor College of Medicine. (2021). *GlyNAC improves multiple defects in aging to boost strength and cognition in older humans.* ScienceDaily. https://www.sciencedaily.com/releases/2021/03/210329122746.htm

Belenky, P., Racette, F. G., Bogan, K. L., McClure, J. M., Smith, J. S., & Brenner, C. (2007). Nicotinamide riboside promotes sir2 silencing and extends lifespan via nrk and urh1/pnp1/meu1 pathways to NAD+. *Cell, 129*(3), 473–484. https://doi.org/10.1016/j.cell.2007.03.024

Belsky, D. W., Huffman, K. M., Pieper, C. F., Shalev, I., & Kraus, W. E. (2017). Change in the rate of biological aging in response to caloric restriction: CALERIE biobank analysis. *The Journals of Gerontology: Series A, 73*(1), 4–10. https://doi.org/10.1093/gerona/glx096

Boukabous, I., Marcotte-Chénard, A., Amamou, T., Boulay, P., Brochu, M., Tessier, D., Dionne, I., & Riesco, E. (2019). Low-volume high-intensity interval training (HIIT) versus moderate-intensity continuous training on body composition, cardiometabolic profile and physical capacity in older women. *Journal of Aging and Physical Activity, 1*(27), 1–34. https://doi.org/10.1123/japa.2018-0309

Bourassa, M. W., Alim, I., Bultman, S. J., & Ratan, R. R. (2016). Butyrate, neuroepigenetics and the gut microbiome: Can a high fiber diet improve brain health? *Neuroscience Letters, 625*(1), 56–63. https://doi.org/10.1016/j.neulet.2016.02.009

Braniste, V., Al-Asmakh, M., Kowal, C., Anuar, F., Abbaspour, A., Toth, M., Korecka, A., Bakocevic, N., Ng, L. G., Kundu, P., Gulyas, B., Halldin, C., Hultenby, K., Nilsson, H., Hebert, H., Volpe, B. T., Diamond, B., & Pettersson, S. (2014). The gut microbiota influences blood-brain barrier permeability in mice. *Science Translational Medicine*, *6*(263), 263ra158–263ra158. https://doi.org/10.1126/scitranslmed.3009759

Buettner, D. (2012). *The Blue Zones: 9 lessons for living longer from the people who've lived the longest*. National Geographic.

Calabrese, E. (2014). Hormesis: a fundamental concept in biology. *Microbial Cell*, *1*(5), 145–149. https://doi.org/10.15698/mic2014.05.145

Cederberg, B. M., & Gray, G. R. (1979). N-acetyl-d-glucosamine binding lectins. A model system for the study of binding specificity. *Analytical Biochemistry*, *99*(1), 221–230. https://doi.org/10.1016/0003-2697(79)90067-8

Center for Food Safety and Applied Nutrition. (2018). *Final determination regarding partially hydrogenated oils*. U.S. Food and Drug Administration. https://www.fda.gov/food/food-additives-petitions/final-determination-regarding-partially-hydrogenated-oils-removing-trans-fat

Center for Disease Control and Prevention. *US Life Expectancy Increased in 2019*. CDC. https://www.cdc.gov/nchs/pressroom/nchs_press_releases/2020/202012.htm

Chen, J., Guo, Y., Gui, Y., & Xu, D. (2018). Physical exercise, gut, gut microbiota, and atherosclerotic cardiovascular diseases. *Lipids in Health and Disease*, *17*(1). https://doi.org/10.1186/s12944-017-0653-9

Chowanadisai, W., Bauerly, K. A., Tchaparian, E., Wong, A., Cortopassi, G. A., & Rucker, R. B. (2010). Pyrroloquinoline quinone stimulates mitochondrial biogenesis through cAMP response element-binding protein phosphorylation and increased PGC-1alpha expression. *The Journal of Biological Chemistry*, *285*(1), 142–152. https://doi.org/10.1074/jbc.M109.030130

Cioffi, F., Senese, R., Lasala, P., Ziello, A., Mazzoli, A., Crescenzo, R., Liverini, G., Lanni, A., Goglia, F., & Iossa, S. (2017). Fructose-Rich diet affects mitochondrial DNA damage and repair in rats. *Nutrients*, *9*(4), 323. https://doi.org/10.3390/nu9040323

Clarke, S. F., Murphy, E. F., O'Sullivan, O., Lucey, A. J., Humphreys, M., Hogan, A., Hayes, P., O'Reilly, M., Jeffery, I. B., Wood-Martin, R., Kerins, D. M., Quigley, E., Ross, R. P., O'Toole, P. W., Molloy, M. G., Falvey, E., Shanahan, F., & Cotter, P. D. (2014). Exercise and associated dietary extremes impact on gut microbial diversity. *Gut*, *63*(12), 1913–1920. https://doi.org/10.1136/gutjnl-2013-306541

Dalla Pellegrina, C., Perbellini, O., Scupoli, M. T., Tomelleri, C., Zanetti, C., Zoccatelli, G., Fusi, M., Peruffo, A., Rizzi, C., & Chignola, R. (2009). Effects of wheat germ agglutinin on human gastrointestinal epithelium: insights from an experimental model of immune/epithelial cell interaction. *Toxicology and Applied Pharmacology, 237*(2), 146–153. https://doi.org/10.1016/j.taap.2009.03.012

Davis, P. A., & Yokoyama, W. (2011). Cinnamon intake lowers fasting blood glucose: Meta-Analysis. *Journal of Medicinal Food, 14*(9), 884–889. https://doi.org/10.1089/jmf.2010.018

Delic, V., Ratliff, W. A., & Citron, B. A. (2021). Sleep deprivation, a link between post-traumatic stress disorder and alzheimer's disease. *Journal of Alzheimer's Disease, 79*(4), 1443–1449. https://doi.org/10.3233/jad-201378

Emek, S. C., Szilagyi, A., Akerlund, H.-E., Albertsson, P.-A., Köhnke, R., Holm, A., & Erlanson-Albertsson, C. (2010). A large scale method for preparation of plant thylakoids for use in body weight regulation. *Preparative Biochemistry & Biotechnology, 40*(1), 13–27. https://doi.org/10.1080/10826060903413057

Evans, C. E. L. (2016). Sugars and health: a review of current evidence and future policy. *Proceedings of the Nutrition Society, 76*(3), 400–407. https://doi.org/10.1017/s0029665116002846

Fight Aging! (2019, May 31). *Does obesity literally accelerate aging?* Fight Aging! https://www.fightaging.org/archives/2019/05/does-obesity-literally-accelerate-aging/

Fleck, S. J., & Falkel, J. E. (1986). Value of resistance training for the reduction of sports injuries. *Sports Medicine, 3*(1), 61–68. https://doi.org/10.2165/00007256-198603010-00006

Foretz, M., Guigas, B., Bertrand, L., Pollak, M., & Viollet, B. (2014). Metformin: From mechanisms of action to therapies. *Cell Metabolism, 20*(6), 953–966. https://doi.org/10.1016/j.cmet.2014.09.018

Foundation Fighting Blindness. (2016). *Nobel-Prize-winning stem-cell researcher delivers keynote at FFB-funded conference in Kyoto.* Foundation Fighting Blindness. https://www.fightingblindness.org/research/nobel-prize-winning-stem-cell-researcher-delivers-keynote-at-ffb-funded-conference-in-kyoto-5027

Franceschi, C. (2008). Inflammaging as a major characteristic of old people: Can it be prevented or cured? *Nutrition Reviews, 65*, S173–S176. https://doi.org/10.1111/j.1753-4887.2007.tb00358.x

Franceschi, C., & Campisi, J. (2014). Chronic inflammation (inflammaging) and its potential contribution to age-associated diseases. *The Journals of*

Gerontology. Series A, Biological Sciences and Medical Sciences, 69 Suppl 1, S4-9. https://doi.org/10.1093/gerona/glu057

Gard, T., Noggle, J. J., Park, C. L., Vago, D. R., & Wilson, A. (2014). Potential self-regulatory mechanisms of yoga for psychological health. *Frontiers in Human Neuroscience, 8*. https://doi.org/10.3389/fnhum.2014.00770

Goldman, B. (2016). *Low-fiber diet may cause irreversible depletion of gut bacteria over generations*. News Center. https://med.stanford.edu/news/all-news/2016/01/low-fiber-diet-may-cause-irreversible-depletion-of-gut-bacteria.html

Gundry, S. R. (2018). *The plant paradox: the hidden dangers in "healthy" foods that cause disease and weight gain*. Harper Wave, An Imprint of HarperCollins Publishers.

Gundry, S. R., & Lipper, J. (2019). *The longevity paradox: how to die young at a ripe old age*. Harper Wave, An Imprint of HarperCollins Publishers.

Harvard Health Publishing. (2019, July 18). *The importance of potassium*. Harvard Health; Harvard Health. https://www.health.harvard.edu/staying-healthy/the-importance-of-potassium

Hill, S. (2021). *What are senolytics? A summary of senotherapeutics*. Lifespan.io. https://www.lifespan.io/news/senolytics/

Hjarlmarsdottir, F. (2019, September 30). *12 foods that are very high in omega-3*. Healthline. https://www.healthline.com/nutrition/12-omega-3-rich-foods#9.-Flax-seeds-(2

Hood, D. A., Memme, J. M., Oliveira, A. N., & Triolo, M. (2019). Maintenance of skeletal muscle mitochondria in health, exercise, and aging. *Annual Review of Physiology, 81*(1), 19–41. https://doi.org/10.1146/annurev-physiol-020518-114310

Hwang, C.-L., Yoo, J.-K., Kim, H.-K., Hwang, M.-H., Handberg, E. M., Petersen, J. W., & Christou, D. D. (2016). Novel all-extremity high-intensity interval training improves aerobic fitness, cardiac function and insulin resistance in healthy older adults. *Experimental Gerontology, 82*, 112–119. https://doi.org/10.1016/j.exger.2016.06.009

Ji, L. L., Gomez-Cabrera, M.-C., & Vina, J. (2006). Exercise and hormesis: activation of cellular antioxidant signaling pathway. *Annals of the New York Academy of Sciences, 1067*, 425–435. https://doi.org/10.1196/annals.1354.061

Jia, G., Su, L., Singhal, S., & Liu, X. (2012). Emerging roles of SIRT6 on telomere maintenance, DNA repair, metabolism and mammalian aging.

Molecular and Cellular Biochemistry, 364(1-2), 345–350. https://doi.org/10.1007/s11010-012-1236-8

Jianqin, S., Leiming, X., Lu, X., Yelland, G. W., Ni, J., & Clarke, A. J. (2015). Effects of milk containing only A2 beta casein versus milk containing both A1 and A2 beta casein proteins on gastrointestinal physiology, symptoms of discomfort, and cognitive behavior of people with self-reported intolerance to traditional cows' milk. *Nutrition Journal, 15*(1). https://doi.org/10.1186/s12937-016-0147-z

Jung, A. P. (2003). The impact of resistance training on distance running performance. *Sports Medicine, 33*(7), 539–552. https://doi.org/10.2165/00007256-200333070-00005

Kagawa, Y. (1978). Impact of westernization on the nutrition of Japanese: Changes in physique, cancer, longevity and centenarians. *Preventive Medicine, 7*(2), 205–217. https://doi.org/10.1016/0091-7435(78)90246-3

Kerr, J. S., Adriaanse, B. A., Greig, N. H., Mattson, M. P., Cader, M. Z., Bohr, V. A., & Fang, E. F. (2017). Mitophagy and Alzheimer's disease: cellular and molecular mechanisms. *Trends in Neurosciences, 40*(3), 151–166. https://doi.org/10.1016/j.tins.2017.01.002

Khaltourina D., Matveyev Y., Alekseev A., Cortese F., Iovita A. Aging Fits the Disease Criteria of the International Classification of Diseases. Mechanisms of Ageing and Development, Article 111230, July 2020.

Khan, N. A., Raine, L. B., Drollette, E. S., Scudder, M. R., Kramer, A. F., & Hillman, C. H. (2014). Dietary fiber is positively associated with cognitive control among prepubertal children. *The Journal of Nutrition, 145*(1), 143–149. https://doi.org/10.3945/jn.114.198457

Kim, J., Yang, G., Kim, Y., Kim, J., & Ha, J. (2016). AMPK activators: mechanisms of action and physiological activities. *Experimental & Molecular Medicine, 48*(4), e224–e224. https://doi.org/10.1038/emm.2016.16

Kim, L. S., Axelrod, L. J., Howard, P., Buratovich, N., & Waters, R. F. (2006). Efficacy of methylsulfonylmethane (MSM) in osteoarthritis pain of the knee: a pilot clinical trial. *Osteoarthritis and Cartilage, 14*(3), 286–294. https://doi.org/10.1016/j.joca.2005.10.003

Kirkland, J. L., & Tchkonia, T. (2020). Senolytic drugs: from discovery to translation. *Journal of Internal Medicine, 288*(5), 518–536. https://doi.org/10.1111/joim.13141

Kretowicz, M., Johnson, R. J., Ishimoto, T., Nakagawa, T., & Manitius, J. (2011). The impact of fructose on renal function and blood pressure.

International Journal of Nephrology, 2011, 315879. https://doi.org/10.4061/2011/315879

LeBlanc, J. G., Milani, C., de Giori, G. S., Sesma, F., van Sinderen, D., & Ventura, M. (2013). Bacteria as vitamin suppliers to their host: a gut microbiota perspective. *Current Opinion in Biotechnology, 24*(2), 160–168. https://doi.org/10.1016/j.copbio.2012.08.005

Lee, S.-H., Lee, J.-H., Lee, H.-Y., & Min, K.-J. (2019). Sirtuin signaling in cellular senescence and aging. *BMB Reports, 52*(1), 24–34. https://pubmed.ncbi.nlm.nih.gov/30526767/

Life Extension Advocacy Foundation. (2021). *What is aging?* Lifespan.io. https://www.lifespan.io/aging-explained/

Litwin H. Physical activity, social network type, and depressive symptoms in late life: an analysis of the data from the National Social Life, health and aging project. Aging Mental Health. 2012; 16(5):608-16

López-Otín, C., Blasco, M. A., Partridge, L., Serrano, M., & Kroemer, G. (2013). The hallmarks of aging. *Cell, 153*(6), 1194–1217. https://doi.org/10.1016/j.cell.2013.05.039

Madzin, A. (2022). *New combination treatment shows promise against dementia.* Lifespan.io. https://www.lifespan.io/news/new-combination-treatment-shows-promise-against-dementia/

Malone, J., & Dadswell, A. (2018). The role of religion, spirituality and/or belief in positive ageing for older adults. *Geriatrics, 3*(2), 28. https://doi.org/10.3390/geriatrics3020028

Manfredi, T. G., Monteiro, M., Lamont, L. S., Singh, M. F., Foldvari, M., White, S., Cosmas, A., & Urso, M. L. (2013). Post-Menopausal effects of resistance training on muscle damage and mitochondria. *Journal of Strength and Conditioning Research / National Strength & Conditioning Association, 27*(2), 556–561. https://doi.org/10.1519/JSC.0b013e318277a1e4

Mattson, M. P., Longo, V. D., & Harvie, M. (2017). Impact of intermittent fasting on health and disease processes. *Ageing Research Reviews, 39,* 46–58. https://doi.org/10.1016/j.arr.2016.10.005

Mavros, Y., Gates, N., Wilson, G. C., Jain, N., Meiklejohn, J., Brodaty, H., Wen, W., Singh, N., Baune, B. T., Suo, C., Baker, M. K., Foroughi, N., Wang, Y., Sachdev, P. S., Valenzuela, M., & Fiatarone Singh, M. A. (2016). Mediation of cognitive function improvements by strength gains after resistance training in older adults with mild cognitive impairment: Outcomes of the study of mental and resistance training. *Journal of the American Geriatrics*

Society, 65(3), 550–559. https://doi.org/10.1111/jgs.14542

Mehmel, M., Jovanović, N., & Spitz, U. (2020). Nicotinamide riboside—the current state of research and therapeutic uses. *Nutrients, 12*(6), 1616. https://doi.org/10.3390/nu12061616

Mercola, J. (2006). *Sweet deception: why Splenda®, Nutrasweet®, and the FDA may be hazardous to your health.* Nelson Books.

Meydani SN, Das S, Pieper CF, Lewis MR, Klein S, Dixit VD, Gupta A, Villareal DT, Bhapkar M, Huang M, Fuss PJ, Roberts SB, Holloszy JO, and Fontana L. (2016). "Long-term calorie restriction inhibits inflammation without impairing cell-mediated immunity: A randomized controlled trial in non-obese humans." *Aging,* 8(7). Published online July 13, 2016.

Minciullo, P. L., Catalano, A., Mandraffino, G., Casciaro, M., Crucitti, A., Maltese, G., Morabito, N., Lasco, A., Gangemi, S., & Basile, G. (2015). Inflammaging and anti-inflammaging: The role of cytokines in extreme longevity. *Archivum Immunologiae et Therapiae Experimentalis, 64*(2), 111–126. https://doi.org/10.1007/s00005-015-0377-3

Miraldi Utz, V., Coussa, R. G., Antaki, F., & Traboulsi, E. I. (2018). Gene therapy for RPE65-related retinal disease. *Ophthalmic Genetics, 39*(6), 671–677. https://doi.org/10.1080/13816810.2018.1533027

Mohammad, A., Thakur, P., Kumar, R., Kaur, S., Saini, R. V., & Saini, A. K. (2019). Biological markers for the effects of yoga as a complementary and alternative medicine. *Journal of Complementary & Integrative Medicine, 16*(1). https://doi.org/10.1515/jcim-2018-0094

Mollica, M. P., Mattace Raso, G., Cavaliere, G., Trinchese, G., De Filippo, C., Aceto, S., Prisco, M., Pirozzi, C., Di Guida, F., Lama, A., Crispino, M., Tronino, D., Di Vaio, P., Berni Canani, R., Calignano, A., & Meli, R. (2017). Butyrate regulates liver mitochondrial function, efficiency, and dynamics in insulin-resistant obese mice. *Diabetes, 66*(5), 1405–1418. https://doi.org/10.2337/db16-0924

Morikawa, M., Okazaki, K., Masuki, S., Kamijo, Y., Yamazaki, T., Gen-no, H., & Nose, H. (2009). Physical fitness and indices of lifestyle-related diseases before and after interval walking training in middle-aged and older males and females. *British Journal of Sports Medicine, 45*(3), 216–224. https://doi.org/10.1136/bjsm.2009.064816

Morris, J. K., Vidoni, E. D., Johnson, D. K., Van Sciver, A., Mahnken, J. D., Honea, R. A., Wilkins, H. M., Brooks, W. M., Billinger, S. A., Swerdlow, R. H., & Burns, J. M. (2017). Aerobic exercise for Alzheimer's disease: A

randomized controlled pilot trial. *PLOS ONE, 12*(2), e0170547. https://doi.
org/10.1371/journal.pone.0170547

Moulis, M., & Vindis, C. (2018). Autophagy in metabolic age-related human
diseases. *Cells, 7*(10), 149. https://doi.org/10.3390/cells7100149

National Center for Complementary and Integrative Health. (2018). *Omega-3
supplements: In depth.* NCCIH. https://www.nccih.nih.gov/health/omega3-
supplements-in-depth

National Institute of Environmental Health Sciences. (2021). *Inflammation.*
National Institute of Environmental Health Sciences. https://www.niehs.
nih.gov/health/topics/conditions/inflammation/index.cfm

National Institute on Aging. (2017). *"SuperAgers" show possible new link between
social engagement, cognitive health.* National Institute on Aging. https://
www.nia.nih.gov/news/superagers-show-possible-new-link-between-
social-engagement-cognitive-health

National Institute on Aging. (2020). *NIA strategic directions 2020-2025.* National
Institute on Aging. https://www.nia.nih.gov/about/aging-strategic-direc
tions-research

National Institute on Aging. (2021). *Vitamins and minerals for older adults.*
National Institute on Aging. https://www.nia.nih.gov/health/vitamins-
and-minerals-older-adults

National Institutes of Health. (2017). *Vitamin K.* Nih.gov. https://ods.od.nih.
gov/factsheets/VitaminK-Consumer/

Okita, K., Ichisaka, T., & Yamanaka, S. (2007). Generation of germline-
competent induced pluripotent stem cells. *Nature, 448*(7151), 313–317.
https://doi.org/10.1038/nature05934

Owen, M. R., Doran, E., & Halestrap, A. P. (2000). Evidence that metformin
exerts its anti-diabetic effects through inhibition of complex 1 of the mitochondrial respiratory chain. *The Biochemical Journal, 348* Pt 3, 607–614.
https://pubmed.ncbi.nlm.nih.gov/10839993/

Pal, H. C., Pearlman, R. L., & Afaq, F. (2016). *Fisetin and its role in chronic
diseases* (S. C. Gupta, S. Prasad, & B. B. Aggarwal, Eds.). Springer Link;
Springer International Publishing. https://link.springer.com/chapter/10.
1007%2F978-3-319-41334-1_10

Patrick J. Skerret, Former Executive Editor, Harvard Health. Is retirement
good for health or bad for it? Harvard Health Blog. December 10 2012

Pauly, T., Lay, J. C., Scott, S. B., & Hoppmann, C. A. (2018). Social relationship
quality buffers negative affective correlates of everyday solitude in an

adult lifespan and an older adult sample. *Psychology and Aging, 33*(5), 728–738. https://doi.org/10.1037/pag0000278

Pérez, V. I., Bokov, A., Remmen, H. V., Mele, J., Ran, Q., Ikeno, Y., & Richardson, A. (2009). Is the oxidative stress theory of aging dead? *Biochimica et Biophysica Acta (BBA)— General Subjects, 1790*(10), 1005–1014. https://doi.org/10.1016/j.bbagen.2009.06.003

Perlmutter, D. (2017). *Brain maker: the power of gut microbes to heal and protect your brain— for life.* Yellow Kite.

Perlmutter, D., & Loberg, K. (2019). *Grain brain: the surprising truth about wheat, carbs, and sugar— your brain's silent killers.* Yellow Kite.

Phillips, B. E., Kelly, B. M., Lilja, M., Ponce-González, J. G., Brogan, R. J., Morris, D. L., Gustafsson, T., Kraus, W. E., Atherton, P. J., Vollaard, N. B. J., Rooyackers, O., & Timmons, J. A. (2017). A practical and time-efficient high-intensity interval training program modifies cardio-metabolic risk factors in adults with risk factors for type II diabetes. *Frontiers in Endocrinology, 8.* https://doi.org/10.3389/fendo.2017.00229

Planque, S. A., Massey, R. J., & Paul, S. (2020). Catalytic antibody (catabody) platform for age-associated amyloid disease: From Heisenberg's uncertainty principle to the verge of medical interventions. *Mechanisms of Ageing and Development, 185,* 111188. https://doi.org/10.1016/j.mad.2019.111188

Popkin, B. M., D'Anci, K. E., & Rosenberg, I. H. (2010). Water, hydration, and health. *Nutrition Reviews, 68*(8), 439–458. https://doi.org/10.1111/j.1753-4887.2010.00304.x

Reginster, J.-Y., Neuprez, A., Lecart, M.-P., Sarlet, N., & Bruyere, O. (2012). Role of glucosamine in the treatment for osteoarthritis. *Rheumatology International, 32*(10), 2959–2967. https://doi.org/10.1007/s00296-012-2416-2

Ridaura, V. K., Faith, J. J., Rey, F. E., Cheng, J., Duncan, A. E., Kau, A. L., Griffin, N. W., Lombard, V., Henrissat, B., Bain, J. R., Muehlbauer, M. J., Ilkayeva, O., Semenkovich, C. F., Funai, K., Hayashi, D. K., Lyle, B. J., Martini, M. C., Ursell, L. K., Clemente, J. C., & Van Treuren, W. (2013). Gut microbiota from twins discordant for obesity modulate metabolism in mice. *Science (New York, N.Y.), 341*(6150), 1241214. https://doi.org/10.1126/science.1241214

Roberts, J. L., & Moreau, R. (2016). Functional properties of spinach (Spinacia oleracea L.) phytochemicals and bioactives. *Food & Function, 7*(8), 3337–3353. https://doi.org/10.1039/c6fo00051g

Ros, M., & Carrascosa, J. M. (2020). Current nutritional and pharmacological anti-aging interventions. *Biochimica et Biophysica Acta (BBA)— Molecular Basis of Disease*, *1866*(3), 165612. https://doi.org/10.1016/j.bbadis.2019.165612

Rose, C. (2018). *Longer daily fasting times improve health and longevity in mice.* National Institute on Aging. https://www.nia.nih.gov/news/longer-daily-fasting-times-improve-health-and-longevity-mice

S, A., D, P., N, P., & Cs, M. (2018, February 1). *Obesity as a risk factor for alzheimer's disease: Weighing the evidence.* Obesity Reviews: An Official Journal of the International Association for the Study of Obesity. https://pubmed.ncbi.nlm.nih.gov/29024348/

Schnell, T., Fuchs, D., & Hefti, R. (2020). Worldview under stress: Preliminary findings on cardiovascular and cortisol stress responses predicted by secularity, religiosity, spirituality, and existential search. *Journal of Religion and Health*, *59*(6), 2969–2989. https://doi.org/10.1007/s10943-020-01008-5

Scientific Research on Maharishi's Transcendental Meditation and TM-Sidhi Program: Collected Papers: Volumes 1-8, MERU Press, MVU Press and MIU Press. Published from: 1977–2020.

SENS Research Foundation. (2021). *AmyloSENS: Removing junk from between cells.* SENS Research Foundation. https://www.sens.org/our-research/intro-to-sens-research/amylosens/

Sharma, S., Agrawal, R. P., Choudhary, M., Jain, S., Goyal, S., & Agarwal, V. (2011). Beneficial effect of chromium supplementation on glucose, HbA1C and lipid variables in individuals with newly onset type-2 diabetes. *Journal of Trace Elements in Medicine and Biology*, *25*(3), 149–153. https://doi.org/10.1016/j.jtemb.2011.03.003

Sherry, C. L., Kim, S. S., Dilger, R. N., Bauer, L. L., Moon, M. L., Tapping, R. I., Fahey, G. C., Tappenden, K. A., & Freund, G. G. (2010). Sickness behavior induced by endotoxin can be mitigated by the dietary soluble fiber, pectin, through up-regulation of IL-4 and Th2 polarization. *Brain, Behavior, and Immunity*, *24*(4), 631–640. https://doi.org/10.1016/j.bbi.2010.01.015

Sinclair, D. (2019). *Lifespan: Why we age, and why we don't have to.* Atria Book.

Smolarek, A. de C., Ferreira, L. H. B., Mascarenhas, L. P. G., McAnulty, S. R., Varela, K. D., Dangui, M. C., de Barros, M. P., Utter, A. C., & Souza-Junior, T. P. (2016). The effects of strength training on cognitive performance in elderly women. *Clinical Interventions in Aging*, *11*, 749–754. https://doi.org/10.2147/CIA.S102126

Stamatakis E, Hamer M, Dunstan DW. Screen-based entertainment time, all-cause mortality, and cardiovascular events: population-based study with ongoing mortality and hospital events follow-up. J Am Coll Cardiol. 2011; 57(3): 292-9.

Swanson, D., Block, R., & Mousa, S. A. (2012). Omega-3 fatty acids EPA and DHA: Health benefits throughout life. *Advances in Nutrition, 3*(1), 1–7. https://doi.org/10.3945/an.111.000893

Tchkonia, T., Zhu, Y., van Deursen, J., Campisi, J., & Kirkland, J. L. (2013). Cellular senescence and the senescent secretory phenotype: therapeutic opportunities. *Journal of Clinical Investigation, 123*(3), 966–972. https://doi.org/10.1172/jci64098

Thomas, D. (2007). The mineral depletion of foods available to us as a nation (1940–2002) – A review of the 6th edition of McCance and Widdowson. *Nutrition and Health, 19*(1-2), 21–55. https://doi.org/10.1177/026010600701900205

Tolahunase, M., Sagar, R., & Dada, R. (2017). Impact of yoga and meditation on cellular aging in apparently healthy individuals: A prospective, open-label single-arm exploratory study. *Oxidative Medicine and Cellular Longevity, 2017*, 1–9. https://doi.org/10.1155/2017/7928981

University of British Columbia. (2018). *Short bursts of intense exercise are a HIIT, even with less active people: Participants find high-intensity interval exercise as enjoyable as traditional exercise.* ScienceDaily. https://www.sciencedaily.com/releases/2018/05/180524141625.htm

Vashum, K. P., McEvoy, M., Shi, Z., Milton, A. H., Islam, M. R., Sibbritt, D., Patterson, A., Byles, J., Loxton, D., & Attia, J. (2013). Is dietary zinc protective for type 2 diabetes? Results from the Australian longitudinal study on women's health. *BMC Endocrine Disorders, 13*(1). https://doi.org/10.1186/1472-6823-13-40

Vedin, I., Cederholm, T., Freund Levi, Y., Basun, H., Garlind, A., Faxén Irving, G., Jönhagen, M. E., Vessby, B., Wahlund, L.-O., & Palmblad, J. (2008). Effects of docosahexaenoic acid–rich n–3 fatty acid supplementation on cytokine release from blood mononuclear leukocytes: the OmegAD study. *The American Journal of Clinical Nutrition, 87*(6), 1616–1622. https://doi.org/10.1093/ajcn/87.6.1616

Wallace, R. K. (2017). *Gut crisis: how diet, probiotics, and friendly bacteria help you lose weight and heal your body and mind.* Dharma Publications.

Wallace, R. K., Dillbeck, M., And, E. J., & Harrington, B. (1982). The effects of the transcendental meditation and tm-sidhi program on the aging process. *International Journal of Neuroscience, 16*(1), 53–58. https://doi.org/10.3109/00207458209147602

Wan, X., & Garg, N. J. (2021). Sirtuin control of mitochondrial dysfunction, oxidative stress, and inflammation in chagas disease models. *Frontiers in Cellular and Infection Microbiology, 11*, 693051. https://doi.org/10.3389/fcimb.2021.693051

Watson, K. (2023, May 24). *Quotes about aging gracefully*. My Caring Plan. https://www.mycaringplan.com/blog/quotes-about-aging-gracefully/

Wei, M., Brandhorst, S., Shelehchi, M., Mirzaei, H., Cheng, C. W., Budniak, J., Groshen, S., Mack, W. J., Guen, E., Di Biase, S., Cohen, P., Morgan, T. E., Dorff, T., Hong, K., Michalsen, A., Laviano, A., & Longo, V. D. (2017). Fasting-mimicking diet and markers/risk factors for aging, diabetes, cancer, and cardiovascular disease. *Science Translational Medicine, 9*(377), eaai8700. https://doi.org/10.1126/scitranslmed.aai8700

Westcott, W. L. (2012). Resistance training is medicine: effects of strength training on health. *Current Sports Medicine Reports, 11*(4), 209–216. https://doi.org/10.1249/JSR.0b013e31825dabb8

Weyh, C., Krüger, K., & Strasser, B. (2020). Physical activity and diet shape the immune system during aging. *Nutrients, 12*(3), 622. https://doi.org/10.3390/nu12030622

Wilber, K. (2001). *A theory of everything: an integral vision for business, politics, science, and spirituality*. Shambhala.

World Health Organization. What is Healthy Ageing? https://www.who.int/ageing/healthy-ageing/en/. Accessed 28 June 2019.

Xiao, B., Sanders, M. J., Carmena, D., Bright, N. J., Haire, L. F., Underwood, E., Patel, B. R., Heath, R. B., Walker, P. A., Hallen, S., Giordanetto, F., Martin, S. R., Carling, D., & Gamblin, S. J. (2013). Structural basis of AMPK regulation by small molecule activators. *Nature Communications, 4*(1), 3017. https://doi.org/10.1038/ncomms4017

Yan, D., Zhang, Y., Liu, L., & Yan, H. (2016). Pesticide exposure and risk of Alzheimer's disease: a systematic review and meta-analysis. *Scientific Reports, 6*. https://doi.org/10.1038/srep32222

Yin, J., Xing, H., & Ye, J. (2008). Efficacy of berberine in patients with type 2 diabetes mellitus. *Metabolism, 57*(5), 712–717. https://doi.org/10.1016/j.metabol.2008.01.013

Yousefzadeh, M. J., Zhu, Y., McGowan, S. J., Angelini, L., Fuhrmann-

Stroissnigg, H., Xu, M., Ling, Y. Y., Melos, K. I., Pirtskhalava, T., Inman, C. L., McGuckian, C., Wade, E. A., Kato, J. I., Grassi, D., Wentworth, M., Burd, C. E., Arriaga, E. A., Ladiges, W. L., Tchkonia, T., & Kirkland, J. L. (2018). Fisetin is a senotherapeutic that extends health and lifespan. *EBioMedicine*, *36*, 18–28. https://doi.org/10.1016/j.ebiom.2018.09.015

Zaccaro, A., Piarulli, A., Laurino, M., Garbella, E., Menicucci, D., Neri, B., & Gemignani, A. (2018). How breath-control can change your life: A systematic review on psycho-physiological correlates of slow breathing. *Frontiers in Human Neuroscience*, *12*(353). https://doi.org/10.3389/fnhum.2018.00353

Zhang, G., Li, J., Purkayastha, S., Tang, Y., Zhang, H., Yin, Y., Li, B., Liu, G., & Cai, D. (2013). Hypothalamic programming of systemic ageing involving IKK-β, NF-ϰB and GnRH. *Nature*, *497*(7448), 211–216. https://doi.org/10.1038/nature12143

Zheng, Z., Bian, Y., Zhang, Y., Ren, G., & Li, G. (2020). Metformin activates AMPK/SIRT1/NF-ϰB pathway and induces mitochondrial dysfunction to drive caspase3/GSDME-mediated cancer cell pyroptosis. *Cell Cycle (Georgetown, Tex.)*, *19*(10), 1089–1104. https://doi.org/10.1080/15384101.2020.1743911

GLOSSARY OF TERMS

Amino acids: Organic compounds that serve as the building blocks of proteins. They are essential for various biological processes and play crucial roles in the structure, function, and regulation of cells and tissues.

AMPK (AMP-activated protein kinase): An enzyme that plays a crucial role in cellular energy metabolism and maintaining energy homeostasis. It is often referred to as the "metabolic master switch" due to its ability to regulate various metabolic pathways and cellular processes.

Antioxidants: Substances that can help protect cells from the damage caused by free radicals. Free radicals are highly reactive molecules that can cause oxidative stress, a process linked to aging and various diseases. Antioxidants neutralize free radicals by donating an electron, thereby stabilizing them, and preventing them from causing damage.

Autophagy: A process by which cells degrade and recycle damaged or dysfunctional cellular components. Autophagy helps maintain cellular homeostasis and has been linked to longevity and anti-aging effects.

Bio-tracking: The monitoring and measurement of various biological parameters and processes within the human body. It involves the use of technology and devices to collect data on physiological, biochemical, or behavioral aspects of an individual's health and well-being. Bio-tracking provides valuable insights into an individual's health status, performance, and overall lifestyle.

Calorie restriction: A dietary intervention that involves reducing calorie intake without malnutrition. Calorie restriction has been shown to extend lifespan and delay the onset of age-related diseases in various organisms.

Cancer: A disease where cells grow uncontrollably. Cancer is a complex and diverse group of diseases characterized by the uncontrolled growth and spread of abnormal cells in the body. It is the leading cause of death worldwide and has a significant impact on individuals, families, and communities.

Cell: Basic structural and functional unit of life. In biology, a cell is the basic structural and functional unit of all living organisms. It is the smallest independently functioning entity that can carry out the essential processes of life.

Chromatins: Strands of DNA wrapped around proteins called histones within the nucleus of the cell. They are highly organized and play a crucial role in regulating gene expression and packaging the genetic information in the cell. There are two types of chromatins: euchromatin, which is open and allows genes to be switched on, and heterochromatin, which is closed and prevents the cell from reading a gene.

Chromosome: A structure into which a cell's DNA is organized. It is held together by proteins. A chromosome is a thread-like structure composed of DNA and proteins found in the nucleus of most cells. It carries genetic information in the form of genes, which are the hereditary units responsible for the transmission of traits from parents to offspring.

Cytokines: Small proteins that serve as signaling molecules in the immune system and other biological processes. They are produced by various cells, including immune cells, and play a crucial role in regulating immune responses, cell communication, inflammation, and other physiological functions.

Deacetylation: The removal of an acetyl group from a molecule, typically through the action of specific enzymes called deacetylases. Acetylation and deacetylation are important post-translational modifications that can regulate the structure, function, and activity of proteins, as well as other biomolecules.

DNA (abbreviation of Deoxyribonucleic Acid): A molecule that encodes information needed for the cell to function or a virus to replicate. DNA is a molecule that carries the genetic instructions for the development, functioning, and reproduction of all living organisms. It is a long, double-stranded molecule composed of nucleotides.

Enzyme: a protein made up of strings of amino acids, that folds into a ball and carries out chemical reactions.

Epigenetic: Changes to a cell's gene expression that arises from non-genetic influences and does not alter the DNA code.

Epigenetic noise: Refers to the random fluctuations or variability in epigenetic marks and gene expression patterns within a population of cells or organisms. It arises from the stochastic nature of these modifications and their dynamic interactions with various cellular processes. Aging is a result, in part, of the propagation of epigenetic noise.

Epigenome: Refers to a collection of chemical modifications and proteins that interact with DNA and regulate gene expression without changing the underlying DNA sequence. It acts as a layer of information that influences how genes are activated or silenced in specific cells.

Euchromatin: Refers to a less condensed and more transcriptionally active form of chromatin within the cell nucleus. It represents the regions of chromatin that are accessible to transcription factors and other regulatory molecules, allowing for gene expression.

Ex-differentiation: The loss of cell identity due to epigenetic noise, which could be associated with aging.

Gene: A gene is a specific segment of DNA that contains the instructions for building proteins that are crucial for the functioning of an organism. It is the fundamental unit of heredity and carries the genetic information that is passed down from parents to offspring.

Gene expression: The process by which information encoded in the genes is used to create functional molecules such as proteins or RNA molecules that perform specific biological functions within a cell or organism.

Gene therapy: The delivery of undamaged DNA to human cells as medical therapy. Gene therapy is a therapeutic approach that aims to treat or prevent diseases by introducing genetic material into a person's cells. It involves modifying or replacing the genetic material to correct or compensate for genetic defects, restore normal cellular function, or introduce new therapeutic functions.

Genome: The entire DNA (deoxyribonucleic acid) sequence of an organism. It includes all the genes, noncoding DNA, and regulatory sequences that determine the structure, function, and characteristics of each organism.

Hayflick limit: Also known as the Hayflick phenomenon or replicative senescence, this refers to the maximum number of times that a normal human cell population can divide before reaching a state of irreversible cell cycle arrest. It was discovered by Dr. Leonard Hayflick in the 1960s while studying human cell cultures.

Histones: The proteins that manage DNA packaging inside the chromosome and allow three feet of DNA to fit inside a cell.

Hormesis: A biological phenomenon in which exposure to low or moderate stress levels or low doses of harmful agents can induce beneficial effects and enhance the organism's resilience and overall health. Often called "good stress," these low levels of stress can trigger cellular processes such as DNA repair, antioxidant production, and activation of protective signaling pathways. Examples of hormetic stressors include exercise, dietary restriction, heat and cold exposure, certain drugs or compounds, and even exposure to low levels of radiation or toxins.

Inflammaging: A term coined by research scientists to put a name to the effects of chronic inflammation, which promotes the development of age-related diseases and the aging process itself.

Intermittent fasting: An eating pattern that involves alternating periods of fasting and eating within a specified time frame. Rather than focusing on what foods to eat, it primarily involves when to eat.

Macrophages: A type of white blood cell that plays a crucial role in the immune system's defense against aging pathogens and foreign substances. They are part of the immune system and are found in various locations throughout the body.

Metformin: A molecule derived from French hellebore plant which is used to treat type II diabetes. It is considered by some to be a longevity medicine.

Mitochondria: As the cell's powerhouse, mitochondria break down nutrients to create energy. This process is called cellular respiration. Mitochondria exist outside of the cell's nucleus and contain their own genome.

Mutation: Genetic mutation refers to a permanent alteration in the DNA sequence of an organism's genome. These changes can occur spontaneously (e.g., faulty DNA copying) or be induced by external factors such as ultraviolet light, radiation, chemicals, or certain viruses. Such variations can cause variety within a species, disease, or be of no consequence.

NAD (Nicotinamide Adenine Nucleotide): Plays a role in energy metabolism, redox reactions, DNA repair, and sirtuin and cellular regulation. NAD decreases as we age; therefore, increasing NAD levels as we get older may help combat aging.

Oxidative stress: Imbalance between the production of reactive oxygen species (ROS) and the body's antioxidant defense system. Oxidative Stress can lead to cellular damage and aging.

Pathogen: A microbe that causes illness.

Polyphenols: A diverse group of natural compounds found in plants. They are characterized by the presence of multiple phenol (aromatic alcohol) rings and have been widely studied for their potential health benefits.

Protein: A string of amino acids folded into a three-dimensional structure that has a role in helping cells to grow, divide, and function.

Rapamycin: Also known as Sirolimus, rapamycin belongs to a class of compounds known as mTOR inhibitors. It has been shown to reduce cellular senescence, extend the lifespans of yeast, worms, flies and mice, enhance glucose sensitivity, and improve glucose homeostasis, thus reducing age related metabolic disorders such as obesity and diabetes. It does, however, have potential side effects that would need to be mitigated if it is to be used as an anti-aging compound.

Resveratrol: A certain compound found in plants, particularly grapes and red wine. Resveratrol has been shown to activate longevity-related pathways and exhibit anti-aging effects in some studies.

Senescent cells: Cellular senescence is a state of permanent growth arrest of old or damaged cells in response to various stressors, including oncogenic, genotoxic, and oxidative stress, radiation and chemotherapeutics, and mitochondrial malfunction. Senescent cells exhibit distinct characteristics including altered gene expression and the secretion of pro-inflammatory molecules. While senescence serves as a protective mechanism, the accumulation of senescent cells can contribute to aging and age-related diseases.

Senolytics: Drugs or compounds that target and selectively eliminate senescent cells. By selectively eliminating senescent cells, senolytics may help reduce chronic inflammation, enhance tissue regeneration, and improve overall tissue function, which may slow down or even reverse aging.

Sirtuins: A family of proteins involved in cellular processes such as DNA repair, metabolism, and stress response. They belong to a group of enzymes that are NAD+-dependent deacetylases that control longevity and need NAD to function. Increasing sirtuin activity helps delay age-related changes.

Stem cells: Undifferentiated cells with the potential to turn into a specialized type of cell. Stem cells decline and dysfunction with age, which interferes with healthy tissue regeneration and repair.

Survival circuit: An ancient biological system at the cellular level which shifts energy away from growth and reproduction toward cellular repair during times of adversity.

Telomeres: Protective caps at the ends of chromosomes that keep the chromosome from fraying, analogous to the aglet at the end of a shoelace. Telomeres shorten with every cell division. This shortening is associated with cellular aging and has been linked to age-related diseases.

Transcription: Refers to the biological process by which genetic information encoded in DNA is converted into RNA molecules. This conversion or transcription can be affected by epigenetic modifications, oxidative stress, and alterations in the activity of transcription factors and co-regulators. These changes can result in dysregulated gene expression patterns leading to cellular dysfunction, tissue degeneration and an increased susceptibility to age-related diseases.

Virus: An infectious entity that can persist only by hijacking a host organism to reproduce itself. Viruses have their own genome but are technically not considered living organisms.

INDEX

M

Made in the USA
Middletown, DE
02 March 2024

50724321R00117